Principles for PERSONAL TRAINERS

88
Essential Rules for Excellence

Teri S. O'Brien, J.D., M.S.

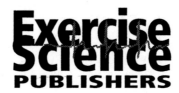

Exercise Science PUBLISHERS

ISBN: 1-58518-326-1
Library of Congress Catalog Card Number: 2001088317

Book layout: Paul Lewis
Cover design: Jennifer Bokelmann, Paul Lewis

Excercise Science Publishers
P.O. Box 1828
Monterey, CA 93942
http://www.healthylearning.com

DEDICATION

To Tom Sattler, who has dedicated his professional life to elevating the professionalism of the fitness industry, and who has been my mentor, my colleague, and best of all, my friend.

CONTENTS

PREFACE

The door to happiness opens outward.
Kierkegaard

People are often astounded to learn that fitness is my second career, especially since my first career, law, required not only an advanced degree, but the passing of the dreaded bar exam. Maybe it's because they realize that, even by the most conservative calculation, I have foregone several hundred thousand dollars in income by changing careers. Maybe they've watched too many episodes of "Ally McBeal" and figure that practicing law means hanging around a unisex bathroom, kickboxing co-workers you don't like and linedancing to Barry White songs in your favorite bar. Whatever the reason, reactions range from an interested "Wow, you really made a switch!" to an almost-sneering "Why would you waste all the schooling?" To the first group, I usually explain that the differences in the two careers are not as dramatic as they think (read on for more on that). As for the second, it's all I can do to patiently remind them that education is never a waste of time, regardless of how you end up using it, which brings me back to the beginning: why I changed careers and how that affects you.

Rarely, if ever, has anyone noticed that I am delighted with my choice, or if they have, they don't say so. I suspect that you understand, though, because you've probably personally experienced the high that comes from seeing someone who had a hard time getting out of a chair walk in his first 5k, and knowing that you had a small part in it. If you haven't, get ready, because if you use the advice in this book, you will become a genuine difference maker in the lives of people you haven't even met.

I mentioned that practicing law and being a personal trainer are more similar than many people think. Does that surprise you? Think about it this way: people come to professionals to solve problems for them by using their knowledge, skill and judgment. If the professional is a lawyer, he uses his knowledge of the statutes, tax code or other applicable law to advise clients about the best way to avoid being sued, paying too many taxes, or in the worst case, staying out of jail. As personal trainers, we use our knowledge of biomechanics, anatomy, and physiology to help people get leaner, stronger and more functional, or to improve their performance in competition. In both cases, clients are relying on our advice and ability to consider all the facts and circumstances and make sure they are in the best possible situation they can be.

Of course, even though thinking of ourselves as professionals on a par with attorneys might make you puff out your chest a bit, that's just the beginning. Having been on both sides of this, I can tell you: no lawyer, with the possible exception of one who frees an innocent person from Death Row, will ever be able to have the positive impact on people that we have every day.

Recently the *Wall Street Journal* reported on the Friendly Supper Club. It began in 1983 in Montgomery, Alabama, at a time of racial strife. Mysteriously, just as tensions were reaching a fever pitch, several dozen Montgomery residents, both black and white, received invitations to dinner from a "Jack Smith." The first month 35 people, driven mostly by curiosity, showed up. The next month, 75. Then 150. Then "Jack Smith," who never revealed his identity, wrote to everyone saying that he was leaving the group on its own, and appointing them all honorary Jack Smiths. The group has been meeting on the first Monday of the month ever since.

One current attendee, a 28-year-old teacher, plans to invite several members of the group to talk to his contemporary issues class. "It will be a great thing for my students to see," he says. "The truth will become flesh and dwell among us."

As personal trainers, we have been given a great gift: the opportunity to make a wonderful truth, the genuine good news about what exercise and a healthful lifestyle can do to dramatically change lives, real for all the people we touch.

INTRODUCTION

I've heard people talk about epiphanies inspired by reflections, as in "I saw the reflection of a really fat person as I walked past a store window, and thought 'how did he let himself get like that?! only to realize, to my shock and horror, that the hideous fat person with the cascading mounds of flesh bursting out of straining sleeves and over the helpless waistband was me! It was then that I decided to turn my life around because I knew that's not the person I wanted to be." In other words, the perception of what was on the outside was at odds with what was known to be on the inside.

Similarly, for years I shuddered when people introduced me as a "personal trainer," because I knew how that label reflected in their eyes: lycra-clad, excessively perky type with a tight rear end and an empty head. Million dollar body, two cent brain. You get the picture. "Wait a second!" I wanted to scream: I'm a health professional! I'm not some dumb bimbette who shows up to count reps and hand someone a pair of dumbbells! That was DEFINITELY not the person I wanted to be, and I wasn't that person! Neither, I suspect, are you. Yet, you know that personal trainers are not equally qualified. There is a wide range of knowledge and experience in our profession, and given some of the bad, if not dangerous, advice that passes for "personal training" in some quarters, I guess we can't blame many members of the lay public for thinking of us as something other than health professionals. After all, the highly-qualified fitness professional and the size-3 hat, size-17 shirt often look the same, at first glance and on the surface.

That's the key: it's a little deeper than the surface, and there's more to it than looking the part. If I've learned one thing in my life, it's this: the difference between schlock and quality, between excellence and mediocrity, and, most important, between success and failure isn't always huge. In fact, sometimes it's downright tiny. Sometimes it's so small in fact that if you aren't looking for it at the time, you'll miss it completely until after the fact, when you'll say "If only. . ." And the "if only" thing won't be a big thing. It will be something that you could have done, probably fairly easily, which would have made a geometric difference in the result. I guess that's why they say "Hindsight is 20/20." If you want to be the best, it's not the devil that's in the details. It's as Mies Van De Rohe, the great architect, said: it's God. That's what this book is about: details. Details that will help you be the best personal trainer you can be. Pearls of wisdom (i.e., principles to be guided by).

Doctors refer to little bits of wisdom they've gathered through experience as "pearls," things that they've learned over the years of treating patients that make them better healers. This book contains things that I've learned in over a decade of working with hundreds of different kinds of clients, things that will make you a more effective, more knowledgeable and more professional personal trainer. Some of them are specific, practical suggestions. Others are on a higher level of abstraction, general attitude-adjustment ideas that I hope will shift your view of your role in your clients' lives and in our profession.

So this book has two objectives: one big and lofty, the other practical and concrete. The lofty goal is to elevate the professionalism of the practitioners in our industry. The practical one, and the one that you're probably going to find most immediately interesting, is to save you time. Why re-invent the wheel, after all? I'm more than happy to share these tips, insights and secrets with you so that you can spend your time on the most important goals of all: becoming one of the outstanding professionals in the field, a sought-after personal training standout with a rabidly-devoted following of clients and a long waiting list of client wannabes, thereby achieving the unsurpassed happiness that only a life of genuine contribution can bring.

#1   *Ask yourself: who is this about?*

I've concluded that for many of us, there is no sweeter sound than the sound of our own voices. If you want your voice to be sweet music to your client as well, you need to remember that you are there for one reason: to serve your client. Now, what are the implications of that fact? Several come to mind. First, you should not be concerned about lecturing your client to prove that you are the smartest person in the room. Your client <u>knows</u> that you're smart. That's why he hired you! The important thing from his perspective isn't only how smart and knowledgeable you are; it's also how well you're able to translate that knowledge into his language, to push his buttons so that he can understand what you're trying to teach him. Otherwise, he'll be standing there thinking "This affects me how?" as in big pile of poop; no pony.

Here's another important thing to remember: your client knows that you're in great shape, and he really doesn't need to see your washboard abs or feel your tight rear-end to prove it to himself. You may think I'm way out in left field with that last one, but I've actually read magazine articles in which "famous," "celebrity" trainers ask their clients do just that! The only body that should be the focus of your attention is your client's, not the other way around. If your goal is to show off your buff bod, consider a career at one of those "tuck-a-buck" bars where you can make scads of money and show off your ass without making one of yourself.

Third, your client has hired you as a professional to help him solve a problem; therefore, in his eyes, you are an authority figure. That may come as a shock to some of you, especially if you are years or even decades younger than some of the people you're training, but it's true. As such, it is extremely inappropriate for you to impose your personal problems on your clients. They don't benefit from helping you recover from a bad breakup, nor does it enhance your reputation to create the impression in their minds of you as a blubbering mass of protoplasm, wallowing in emotional pain. Take your problems to your minister, your therapist, your friends, your mother, anyone but your clients! Ditto the stories about the weekend binge and the subsequent hangover. Thanks for sharing, Sparky, but we're not interested!

One phrase that will keep you on track: it's not about you, it's about them. I'm sure you've all had the experience of having a professor who obviously knew a great deal. Maybe he had several shelves of books published and pages and pages of articles and scholarly journals and credentials up the wazoo and, yet, when he stood up in front of you, it was obvious that he knew a lot. You just didn't know what it had to do with you. Big pile of poop: no pony.

I've seen trainers like that. They are so busy showing off and proving that they are the smartest people in the room, that the client is almost an afterthought. Unfortunately, when I watch them, another phrase to remember springs to mind: Empty barrels make the most noise. Showing off how much you know, especially in an excessively loud tone of voice, is not what personal training is about.

> **Principle #1: Keep repeating this phrase to yourself: It's not about me; it's about him (or her).**

 But I don't even know how to operate an overhead projector!

Personal trainers need to keep in mind that a big part of their job is education. At least it should be. We need to be very much in the teach-a-man-to-fish-and-you-feed-him-for-lifetime frame of mind. Your goal should be to teach your client what he needs to know to be his best, and to help him internalize these behaviors. Sometimes I think that trainers are afraid to empower their clients, thinking that if they don't create dependency, their clients won't "need" them anymore. The exact opposite is true: the more you teach your clients about what you're doing and why, the more loyal they will become, and the more eager they will be to see you because they know that after seeing you they will know things that they didn't know before. They will also rave about you to all of their friends, speaking of you in glowing terms more befitting Gandhi than you or any other mere mortal.

Think about the great teachers you've had. They impart knowledge seemingly by osmosis. They are inspiring. They are life-long learners. Most of all, they are focused, not on themselves, but on their students.

- Good teachers are organized.
- Good teachers are prepared.
- Good teachers are not lazy.
- Good teachers don't shrink from the challenge of working with the hard-to-reach, and the same goes for good personal trainers. Of course, it's harder to posture and show how smart you are to someone who may not know the first thing about your subject.

Recently, I was working out, minding my own business, when I was approached by one of the club's trainers, who wanted to discuss my form on the lat pulldown. While we were debating the merits of one additional micron of range of motion, and mere steps away from us, was an elderly, obese woman practically riding another lat pulldown like a teeter-totter. She'd jerk the bar down to the top of her thighs, then fly off the seat as the weight stack crashed down loudly. After he got done chatting me up, he strolled right past her without saying a word. Was that because she was invisible to him? Was it because it's more enjoyable to talk to someone who knows terms like "lat" and "range of motion?" I have no idea what was in his head—I could say "not much," but why state the obvious?

It's always easier to preach to the converted, and no doubt more gratifying to your ego to demonstrate your vast body of knowledge to someone who can appreciate it, but ask yourself "how can I have the most impact?" That answer is also obvious.

Of course, it's primarily for our clients that we want to be teachers, but that doesn't mean there's nothing in it for us. Sometimes if you think of a person's life it's easy to become a bit discouraged. After all, it may seem that each of us has about as much impact as a hand swishing around in a bucket of water: once the hand pulls out, there is no evidence of its having been there. Perhaps that's why you hear people say so often that they want to "make a difference." The teaching function of personal training makes it possible for you to do just that, which is why it is one of the most satisfying parts of the job. It's the part that gives you the opportunity to make a lifelong contribution to the lives of the people you train. Rocket scientist—yes, he really was a rocket scientist—Wernher von Braun said "All one can really leave one's children is what's inside their heads. Education, in other words, and not earthly possessions is the ultimate legacy, the only thing that cannot be taken away." Even though they may not be children, the same sentiment applies to our clients. Years after they have left our able tutelage, their lives will be enriched by the things that we teach them.

Principle #2: Think of yourself as a teacher.

 ### *God gave you two ears and one mouth for a reason.*

You can't learn anything while you're talking, and if you don't learn what concerns your client, you don't have a prayer of effectively coaching him. So you have to listen. It's always so easy to get distracted. Studies show people can think a lot faster than they can talk, so it might seem natural for you to be thinking about why you don't like peanut butter or whether three blades really *are* better than two while your client is telling you what he did over the weekend. It might *seem* natural, but you can't let it be.

And notice that I said you need to *listen*, which is something more than hearing. It's hearing plus understanding, which is why listening is an active process, or should be. Let me illustrate with an example. A frequent caller to my radio program and I were talking on the air. He wanted some information that I had given out on a recent show, but that he hadn't written down. I told him that it was posted on my web page, and asked him if he knew the address. It turns out that he doesn't use the Internet yet, so he replied "I hear it all the time, but since it doesn't apply to me, I don't really listen." You can hear something a million times, but if you don't think it applies to you, you won't really listen in that active connected way we're talking about.

Everything your client says applies to you, and should be important to you. So how can you be an effective listener? There are three components to effective listening: mirroring, validating and empathizing.

Mirroring- Think of all the trouble that could be avoided if people didn't assume they knew what people mean, mentally (God forbid, even literally) finishing their sentences without letting them finish.

Sometimes I catch my husband trying to "fill in" gaps in my brilliant discourses. He figures he's heard my babbling for so many years, he knows what I'm going to say before I say it, so when he doesn't hear *exactly* what I say, he's got a pretty good idea. Sometimes he's right, but when he's not, what we have is a failure to communicate, which makes me unhappy. As I always say, "When momma ain't happy, ain't nobody happy." In the context of your relationship with your client, you can substitute the word "client" for "momma," and you'll have a pretty good idea of the problems inherent in not making sure you understand precisely what your client is saying.

You can avoid this pitfall by using mirroring, repeating the statement to demonstrate that you understand what the speaker means. When you use mirroring, you dramatically reduce the risk of misunderstandings. You have a lot fewer of those "Who's on first?" conversations. Most important, you genuinely communicate.

When you mirror your client's statements, choose your words carefully. Make sure that you consider your client's background and style of speaking and model your statements along those lines. For example, if your client has an extensive vocabulary, don't hesitate to throw in a $5 word in your restatement of his thought. On the other hand, be careful not to confuse the issue. Your goal is understanding, not trying to prove that you got a thesaurus for Christmas.

Validating. When you think about it, feelings are the ultimate subjective things, so it should always be possible for you to validate what you hear. People get really hung up on this, though, I think because they are confused about the meaning of the verb "to validate." Contrary to popular belief, validating does not necessarily mean agreeing. Rather, it means stating that you understand how someone *in the speaker's position* might think or feel that way. As in saying, "I guess I never would slash someone in the face with a straight razor because she had 16 items in the '10 items or fewer' line in the grocery store, but I understand that you must have been very angry," while thinking "this one's a real wackjob!"

Where your clients are concerned, it will be much easier. For example, you might hate cats, but if your client's cat dies, you should be able to honestly say "You must feel terrible. I know Fluffy meant a lot to you." Remember it's not about you.

Empathizing: The final step is expressing compassion with the speaker's feelings about the situation he or she described. Once again, this is the time for putting yourself in your client's place. It might take some effort, but the beneficial effects on your relationship with your client make it well worth it.

Principle #3: Understand and practice the components of effective listening.

 What Mies Van de Rohe knew and you need to.

Woody Allen said that eighty percent of success is showing up. If only it were that easy: just showing up and looking the part, wearing your spandex or your warmups and posing on the equipment. Despite what you may see in your local gym, that's not enough. The difference between professional personal trainers and glorified spotters, meddling gym rats, and leg warmer models is that professionals know the details that make all the difference in a client's health, happiness and success.

What makes a really great experience? If you take a step back and consider peak experiences, I think you will realize that often the difference between the really great times and the just so-so are little things. Similarly, if you think about situations that leave you with a negative impression, sometimes they don't suck because of any big thing: think of the beautiful hotel suite with a hair in the sink, the gorgeous cover girl with a piece of spinach between her teeth.

In the context of your programs and your dealings with your clients, the best is the enemy of the good; that is, if you neglect doing the things that raise the bar of service and professionalism, your clients will notice, and they will feel short-changed. Worst case scenario: they start looking around for someone who *doesn't* forget the little things.

I had a secretary once, who soon became an ex-secretary, not only because of the incident I am about to describe, but rather because of a series of screw-ups like this. I had to go to San Francisco on business, and as was customary, she made the airline reservations. Imagine my shock and horror to arrive at the San Francisco airport prepared to return home, only to discover that my return flight was already boarding. In Oakland. To quote the late Dorothy Parker, "there is no there there" Oakland. No kidding. There are two airports in the Bay area, and it was her job to know that. It was a detail, a matter of three letters designating an airport, but it caused me to waste an entire day, not to mention probably shortened my life due to the stress!

Always think about the little things that will make workouts more effective and more enjoyable for your clients. Otherwise, the excellence plane will be leaving and you won't be on it.

> ### Principle #4: God is in the details, and so is being your best.

 ### Screaming, barking and other kennel behaviors

Have you noticed that our profession has had a tough time gaining credibility? Maybe you've even mumbled under your breath when someone asked you what you do for a living. Maybe you've even made something up, something more prestigious like "washroom attendant." Maybe your parents tell relatives that you're in prison, but with good behavior. . . OK, I'm exaggerating, but it has been an uphill battle getting the general public to understand that we are health professionals, not dumb muscleheads and silicone-injected bimbos. I think that one of our biggest obstacles to gaining the credibility that many of us deserve is the stereotype of the personal trainer as a cross between a drill instructor and the Marquis de Sade. Consider by contrast the quiet dignity and authority exuded by a respected doctor or lawyer, and you'll understand why many members of the public think personal trainers are well-built, loud-mouthed buffoons.

Some of us actually enjoy this reputation. I have heard dozens of stories of personal trainers taking apparent sadistic glee in pushing their clients to the brink of, if not a stroke or MI, nausea and severe exhaustion, as if this sort of counter-productive torture marks them as great trainers. They seem to think that their professional standing will improve in direct proportion to number of people who fear the pain and suffering a workout with them will entail. People who labor under this mistaken belief do themselves and their clients a tremendous disservice. Even worse, they damage our entire profession in the eyes of the public. Any moron can yell and scream at someone, and many do. It doesn't take any knowledge or ability to push someone to the brink. A coach encourages and motivates with the authentic authority that flows from his or her knowledge, character and communication skills, and the respect that he or she cannot help but command. He or she understands the art and science of individualized program design. There is no substitute for this kind of genuine ability. Think of that old commercial for the stock brokerage firm: When you know your stuff, you don't have to raise your voice to get people to listen.

> **Principle #5: Lose the drill instructor act.**

The case of the popular restaurant:

Submitted for your approval: two alternative realities. In the first, you and your significant other eagerly arrive at a popular new restaurant. You can't wait to sample the cuisine and atmosphere that have all the critics and many of your friends raving about this place. "Two, please, non-smoking," you tell the hostess. "And how long is the wait?" She chews on her pencil and furrows her brow while she looks down at her clipboard. "Thirty minutes," she says. OK. So you wait in the bar. At 20 minutes, you're starting to get very antsy. At 31, you're looking at your watch every 10 seconds and muttering under your breath. At 35, you're really hating this place, and you don't care if the Rolling Stones serve your dinner to you while the Rockettes perform at your table: you're steamed.

In the parallel universe, you arrive at an identical restaurant, about which you've also heard wonderful things. You approach an identical hostess stand and say to an identical hostess "Two, please, non-smoking." "And how long is the wait?" "Thirty minutes," she says. You and your date go to the bar. At 20 minutes, you're starting to get very antsy. At 25, you see the hostess, who has come into the bar to escort you to your waiting table. You walk to your table, happily anticipating a terrific meal.

Now, in both cases, the hostess was mistaken in her estimate of when your table would be ready by 5 minutes, but in the first case, you are extremely unhappy, while in the latter, you're delighted.

Do you see the difference? Your expectation creates your reaction. In the case of your client, you should keep this scenario in mind.

I'm convinced that the medical profession learned this lesson long ago. Doctors seem to always overstate the severity of illnesses, then when patients recover sooner than expected, they look like geniuses!

> **Principle #6: Underpromise and overdeliver.**

#7 *You think you want lots of clients, but that's not what you really want.*

Sometimes people call us for personal training and they are disappointed to learn that we require new clients to sign up for a minimum of 8 sessions. It's simply not profitable to see a new client for one or two times. If you think about it, the reasons should be obvious. From your standpoint, personal training service is like a mortgage: the costs are front-loaded. The most obvious cost of working with a new client is the cost of signing him up in the form of dollars spent for marketing and advertising, but consider the following hidden costs: *Set-up issues—location, pets, children, and equipment.*

These issues are less of a concern for those who work in gyms or clubs, but for in-home trainers, they are huge. Working with a new client is like a first date. First, you've got to find the place, which may or may not be easy when you've never been there before. Then you've got to deal with whatever you find when you get there. Recently I appeared in a local news fitness series. For the segment on "Choosing a Personal Trainer," the TV mavens wanted to shoot me in action with a client in the client's home. After phoning around to some of my favorite clients, I located what I thought would be perfect: a beautiful, fully-equipped home gym complete with track-lighting, Olympic squat rack, top-of-the-line multi-station machine and a full rack of chrome dumbbells. The reporter working on the piece was very impressed, but she said "this might be almost too nice." I explained to her that in my experience we had basically two choices: a showplace like the one we were in, or a dark, damp basement with piles of laundry and old magazines surrounding a lone bench and chair with a hodgepodge of garage sale equipment on the floor (sort of like my home workout area, sadly). And that's what you might find on your first visit to a client's house. Or you might find a room that looks like a Toys R Us after a bomb goes off with one of those rubber-band-based resistance machines propped up against the wall. (Those are *REAL* easy to deal with, let me tell you: it only takes about two hours to change the amount of resistance between exercises.) Whatever it is, the first time you go there it will be much more difficult and time-consuming to deal with than the next time, and much much more difficult than the 200th time.

So will the pets you might find. Ever have to keep a dog from choking? I have, right in the middle of a workout. Once I stood by helplessly while a client broke up a fight between her two huge dogs, one a German Shepherd, one a Newfoundland. Are you allergic to cats? If so, it might be helpful to know that your new client has twelve who all just *LOVE* to snuggle.

Children present a challenge, too. As you probably realize, you need to make sure they stay out of harm's way so they don't sustain or cause an injury to themselves or your client. The first time you arrive at the house you'll need to explain the ground rules. All of these issues involve additional time and effort on your part, time and effort that you won't have to spend with standing clients.

Lost effectiveness

If you're like me, one of the things you enjoy most about working in fitness is the ability to have an impact on the health and wellness of your clients. Obviously, if you work with someone consistently for a long time, you'll be able to have a greater impact.

Lost referrals

Long-time clients are satisfied clients, and satisfied clients tend to tell their friends and acquaintances how wonderful you are.

No buzz

One of your goals should be to get a reputation, and not the kind our mothers warned us against. You want a reputation as "the best trainer in Anytown, U.S.A," or if Anytown is large, "the best trainer on the north side of Anytown." You get the idea. You want people to think "great personal trainer" and immediately think of you. If you don't have lots of satisfied (as in long-term) clients, you'll have a tough time getting there.

Bottom line: what you really want is a book of <u>standing</u> clients that you see on an ongoing basis. You want to see the same people week after week for as long as possible.

Principle #7: Understand the hidden costs of client turnover.

 Only a life lived for others is worth living. __*Albert Einstein*

Personal training is a very rewarding career, but at times the rewards can get lost in the physical and emotional exhaustion that is often the result of a job that is part furniture mover, part counselor, part conscience and part mother bear up on her hind legs defending her charges. Sometimes you just feel fried, don't you? Between the stress of traffic, crazy schedules, and fatigue, it's no wonder!

So there'll be times when you worry that you're going to fall asleep in traffic and end up as the filling in a semi-truck sandwich, or when you think that if you have to act perky and cheerful one more day when you have a splitting headache, you'll put someone's head through a wall. It's during those times that you need to shift your attention and listen to different voices.

You know that we all have several voices in our heads at any given time competing for our attention. One voice is the "I'm exhausted and I don't want to talk to anyone for at least a week" voice that is often screaming the loudest at you when you get home at the end of a long training day. But there are other voices, such as the one that says "wow—isn't it great the way that she was able to finish that whole 5 k when a year ago she couldn't even walk around the block!" And then the thrilling revelation, "I was a part of that!!" Suddenly you don't feel so tired after all.

I used to notice that no matter how long the day, when I was with a client, I didn't feel tired. The minute I walked in the door at home, I'd collapse literally and figuratively like a ragdoll. What was up with that? I finally realized that when I was with a client I was so absorbed in what we were trying to accomplish together that I didn't even notice how tired I was. In other words, I was so happy I didn't know how miserable I was!

> **Principle #8: Keep reminding yourself of why you got into the fitness profession in the first place.**

 ### There's no one else exactly like you.

Or any of your clients either. Every one of us is unique and special. Sure, you know that, right? We all know that, and we pay lip service to it almost every day, but I'm not sure that we connect with it in any meaningful way. We're all rushing from pillar to post every day, focused on our own agendas, not realizing what we're missing not getting to know all the special people we shove aside trying to get where we're going.

In context of your relationship with your clients, you need to get to know each of them as people. You need to have what I like to call a Level 3 relationship with him. Let me explain what I mean.

I like to think of relationships as if they were three-story buildings. Within each of the three levels, there's some room to move around: there are cubicles and there are corner offices, but for our purposes you simply need to understand the basic three levels.

Level #1

This is your basic superficial interaction, the sort of relationship you have with the cashier at the grocery store that you see every week or the postal worker who delivers your mail. It's more than mere passing acquaintance, but not much. You'll be at this level with clients for a while. The precise amount of time varies depending on how often you see a client, and how much the two of you have in common. It will also depend in large part on your skills as a listener and communicator. I would hope that, assuming you see a client at least once a week, it wouldn't be more than 3 or 4 weeks.

Level #2

Level 2 is your basic good working relationship. It's the relationship you have with your lawyer and your accountant, for example. You know each other on more than a superficial level, and you've learned enough about each other to know that you can work well together to accomplish shared objectives. When you reach Level 2 with your client, you have begun to learn more about his individual preferences, especially his exercise preferences. You are also beginning to gain some insight into your client's personal and work life, and the special challenges that they cause in his life day-to-day. While it's possible to have a long-term trainer-client relationship at Level 2, such a relationship pales in intensity and, therefore, effectiveness, with a Level 3 relationship.

Level #3

Now you're cooking. When you reach Level 3, you know not only all the Level 2 stuff, but also what TV shows they stay home to watch, their kids' birthdays, and the name of the jerk at work that they'd like to strangle. You have become a trusted confidant and, at least as far as the client is concerned, a friend. (I say "as far as they're concerned" because you should still keep your personal problems to yourself. Level 3 is like a close, but one-way, friendship.)

Why is it important to get to Level 3? The answer: so that you can give your client exactly what he needs when he needs it.

Yogi Berra said "You can observe a lot by watching." Learn to read physical cues because sometimes they will conflict with the words coming out of your client's mouth. Can't you imagine the clerk at the grocery store keeling over dead if, in response to his "How are you?" you really told him? Of course. We know that we are supposed to respond with the expected, as in, politically-correct answer: "Fine." Are you sure? If you ask your client how he is, and she says "fine," but she looks like she's ready to burst into tears, you should be in tune with that. If you're at Level 3, you will be the one person she'll feel comfortable talking to, and if need be, crying in front of.

Understanding your client's uniqueness means knowing when to push your client and when to back off. You'll know because you'll know something about your client's energy checking account and his schedule. You'll know because you *know* your client. Personal training, remember, must be personal.

Principle #9: Appreciate the uniqueness of every client.

#10 *Because I'm a professional, dammit!!*

Once when I was practicing law, I went to a negotiation with a client. The guy on the other side was a stereotypical real estate developer type, and rather up in years. We walked in, and he said to my client "how dare you have a lawyer who looks like this? My lawyer looks like an old douche bag!" I suppose I could have gotten all huffy and acted like I was being sexually harassed, but I just smiled my best Miss America smile, knowing my client would be at a distinct advantage. It was about him, after all.

Why do so many personal trainers persist in embracing the mentality that being a great trainer means pushing people until they have a stroke? Aside from the matter of seeing a piece of paper with the word "defendant" on it, and more horrifying, with your name preceding the word "defendant"—YIKES!, I think there's another reason we need to rethink some of this posturing. Some of the personal trainers that I observe seem to enjoy this power trip stuff a little bit too much.

Why are we so rigid about giving body fat and similar tests? We might tell ourselves that the reason is that we want to evaluate our clients' fitness for their benefit, and I'm sure that sometimes that is the case. But is there really any benefit in trying to measure the body fat of a 300-pound woman with mounds of flesh bursting out of every sleeve and cascading over her waistband? That's not going to tell you anything, other than how much flab you can jam into calipers without breaking them. The obsessive need to rigidly adhere to protocol is a way of taking yourself WAY too seriously: you must have a body fat test at 0600 hours every six weeks. Why? Because I AM A PROFESSIONAL, DAMN IT!! This is my job!!

Hold your horses there, partner. If you take your job seriously, you need to know when to make exceptions to your standard operating procedures. You know that your real job is to help your client reach his goals, which is sometimes a matter of using all your fancy knowledge to do physical tests, but always a matter of giving your client what he needs when he needs it.

> **Principle #10: Take your job, but not yourself, seriously.**

#11   *Dig this hole exactly three feet in diameter. Pile the dirt up close by. Fill it up again.*

As a corporate refugee, I've had lots of opportunity to see many kinds of managers. Some of them are just that: managers. Some of them are managers plus. They are leaders. I'll explain the difference in a minute, and trust me, you'll understand why this is and should be important to you.

This point is related to Principle #10 because if you are taking your job seriously by trying to do what's best for your client, you'll realize that there is a difference between doing the right thing and doing things right. "Doing things right" means that you are a master of locating the body landmarks involved in doing a body composition test. You are a wizard with the calipers. No one can instruct a beginner in the proper way to do a squat better than you can. You dream of the Karvonen formula and wake up chanting "VO2 reserve." These technical things are all important. In fact, they are essential to know. I don't mean to suggest that they are not. It's just that they are Step 2, and you want to begin with Step 1.

Huh? Yes. You see, as important as it is to master the technical skills of your profession, you need to start out with a vision of what you want to accomplish, and THEN, and ONLY THEN, figure out which of the technical skills and other tools in your bag of tricks are appropriate to use to best reach that objective. That's the "doing the right thing" part.

If you don't take a step back and think about where you want to help your client go, you are like the "make work" road crew boss, who supervises the digging and re-filling of holes: he doesn't know why he does it, but he does it better than anyone!

> **Principle #11: Understand the difference between doing the right thing and doing things right.**

 #12   *Enthusiasm is contagious: be a carrier!*

Entire books have been written on the subject of body language, and that's no surprise: studies have shown that over half of the information we communicate to others is communicated by our body language. It has even become a pop psych cliché: "his body language wasn't very receptive." "I could tell by her body language that she was giving off a buy signal." We've all heard people say things like this. Heck, you've probably said them yourself. Would it come as a surprise to think that perhaps people say similar things about you? And when they do, do they say things like "What happened to her: did her dog die, her truck breakdown and her mama go back to prison?" Ok, maybe that was a country song, but you get the point. They probably don't say that to your face, but you don't even want them thinking it. Instead, you want your body language to convey alacrity for the task at hand, even if you've got a 3-day migraine in progress. That is one of the biggest challenges of being a personal trainer: there are doubtlessly going to be days when you just don't feel like acting perky and enthusiastic. On those days, you think that if you have to act interested in one more story about somebody's cleaning lady, you're going to jump out the window! Doesn't matter, Sparky. You've got to suck it up and act as you always do, as if your very next breath depends on every word your client says. Most important, you have to appear as if it does because remember most of what we communicate, we communicate non-verbally.

So lift your rib cage and pull your shoulder blades back. You've got some coaching to do.

Principle #12: Make sure that your attitude and body language reflect enthusiasm.

 Schedule Hell.

If you were looking for a job, would you ask a homeless guy? Of course not! He doesn't have enough money to buy his own lunch, let alone give you a job. What he does have is all the time in the world. Where is he going, after all?

On the other hand, the high achievers in our society are constantly juggling the hundreds of balls that they have in the air. There are never enough hours in the day. This is the world most of our clients live in. They have many demands on their time, and these demands are constantly changing. You've got to be ready for this fact, and to the extent possible, try to stay ahead of it.

In a service business, an extremely important part of good customer service is flexibility. Let's say that you have a standing client who always works out at 5:30 PM on Wednesdays. If she has to go out of town on business and can't fit that workout in then, you should do your damnedest to find another spot for her. Remember: one of your goals is to minimize client turnover, and the best way to do that is to bend over backwards to accommodate your clients. The idea is that you should establish some working hours for yourself, but be prepared to be flexible, especially to accommodate good, standing clients.

Equally important is the perception of flexibility. Never make it seem that your client is inconveniencing you or making your life tough, even if the thought enters your mind. Some clients don't have the best people skills, and when they ask you to change their schedules, they don't always have the tact and diplomacy of a UN delegate. That doesn't matter. You need to treat these requests with a smile. Remember, you are in business to serve your clients, and they have to be able to see, smell, and feel that fact. It has to be reflected in your every word, deed and phone call. Sometimes we think that if we're on the phone, people can't tell if we're rolling our eyes and otherwise expressing sarcasm or disgust, but you know from personal experience that that's not true. Just as you can tell when someone is annoyed with you for making a request, so can they.

To be able to change the day and time of a standing appointment, you need to have some free hours in your schedule every day, which is another reason not to book every free minute with client sessions. Not only will you get burned out fast, you won't be able to accommodate any requests to change days or times.

Another thing you may not have thought of: there may be a time when you need a little flexibility from a client. There have been many times when I have, for example, when I needed to out of town to make some video tapes or to attend a professional meeting. When you ask a client to do you the favor of changing your schedule—and that's how you should put it—and he agrees to do so, be sure to show your appreciation. I have a client, let's call her May, who is without a doubt one of the nicest people on the planet, but one thing that gets her hackles up is being dissed, especially when it comes to her schedule. When someone behaves as if he or she is *telling* May *about*, not *asking* her *for*, a schedule change, the heart of this charming, accommodating person turns to stone: she wouldn't change that schedule now at gunpoint, even if it really is no problem for her. It's the principle of the thing. She's not going to be dissed. So ask, don't tell, when you are the one initiating the schedule change.

Principle #13: Be flexible enough to accommodate client requests.

 Say it loud. Say it proud.

It's so tempting when you start out to go through a thought process similar to this: "I'm just starting out in this business and I need to get some clients! What's the quickest way to get clients. . . mmm. . .I could offer to wash their windows for free if they hire me as a personal trainer. . . I could give away a free treadmill to every client who signs up. . .wait a second, I can't afford that!!. . .that's it—affordable. I'll make myself really affordable!" So, you research your service area and decide to set your hourly rate at $10 lower than the going rate. Sure enough, before you know it, you are booked solid. After all, you are like the stuff in the newspaper coupon insert every week—you are a bargain! All is well for a while until one day you are slapped up the side of the head by a realization: you are physically and emotionally exhausted. Not only that, you are starting to resent the people you can least afford to resent: your beloved clients! Yikes—how did this happen?! Actually, it was quite predictable. You see, you forgot a couple of key things: first, that personal training can be an extremely demanding and draining job. (I think I warned you about that, but some things you can only learn by doing, I guess.) The second thing you forgot is that you don't bill every hour that you work. You bill only for the hour that you are there, but what about the time you spend preparing workouts, looking up information, phoning around for referrals and the gazillion other things that we do for clients? That takes time, and time is your stock-in-trade. You look around and you see that you are busting your butt and barely making ends meet! Definitely not a feel good. Now think about it: if you are not only exhausted all the time but also feel that you are not earning what you deserve to earn compared with other people doing the same job, how enthusiastic are you going to be about working with clients? When you lose your enthusiasm for working with clients, two things happen, both of which are bad: (1) you go through the motions during sessions, and your clients get even more bored with you than you are with yourself, and (2) you end up having to confront all your clients with a rate increase. Anytime you raise rates, you may lose at least some clients. When that happens, you have a choice: you can replace the ones that you lose, and therefore replace the income that they provided, or live with less income. Neither of these alternatives is very appealing.

I think that the reason so many personal trainers undervalue their service, and therefore underprice themselves, is fear, fear that they won't find any clients willing to pay them the $40, $50 or $60 dollars an hour that they are worth. It's natural to be a little nervous when you first start out, but have confidence. You know that you are worth it, and if you don't know that, you've got no business masquerading as a professional. So, since you know it, say it loud, say it proud. We all know that the laws of supply and demand dictate that commodities in limited supply command a higher price. You are selling your time, of which there is a limited supply.

I'm warning you: if you don't follow my advice on this one, you will find yourself in the unenviable position of having to present all of your clients with a rate increase, a disruptive event under the best of circumstances. (Any time you have to switch from talking about your client's goals to talking about money, it's disruptive.) You may even lose some clients, or at least create a bad taste in their mouths. So do your homework, and set fair and reasonable rates based on your experience, education and the market in your area.

> **Principle #14: Don't undervalue (and therefore underprice) your service.**

 #15   *Can't anyone there take a *&^%$## message?!*

Have you ever seen that movie, "The King of Comedy?" Robert DeNiro plays an emotionally disturbed man, Rupert Pupkin, who stalks a late-night talk show host played by Jerry Lewis. Rupert fantasizes about being a famous talk show host like Jerry, and his fantasies aren't limited to daydreams. He constructs his own version of the talk show set in his basement, complete with life-size cardboard cutouts of celebrity guests. One of his favorite activities is to sit in the host's chair and pretend to interview these cardboard "guests." Often when he is in the middle of acting out the role of host, you hear his mother off-camera yelling to him "Rupert, you're going to miss the bus," causing him to scream back at the top of his lungs "MAAA! I'm busy down here!" This yelling—"MAAA!—is incredibly grating and adds to the comic aspect of the film.

In real life, though, and when you run your business, it won't be funny when potential clients call, if they hear something like "MAAA!!" when they call and ask for you.

Then there's kids answering the phone. Sometimes I think people, understandably, because they find their children so cute, forget how annoying it is to call someone and have a child answer the phone. If you're calling a business, the irritation factor goes up geometrically.

Remember that clients come to us to solve a problem. If you call a number looking for someone to solve a problem, among the things that you'll probably find REALLY annoying are the following:

- kids answering the phone and barely being able to carry on anything resembling an intelligent conversation
- parents, roommates or spouses who can't find a pencil and don't know when you're coming home

Once I called a client who lives with her parents. I had to endure about 15 minutes of "oh, hold on, I can't find a pencil," getting more irritated by the second.

I have a friend who is the world's biggest technophobe. (You know who you are, Matt.) I don't know if he's gotten over his fear of ATM machine's yet, but he doesn't have a computer. Well, he has one that his dad gave him, but he's afraid to learn to use it. His one concession to modern communication is a fax machine. Recently he went away on a trip, and I tried about 700 times to send him a fax. The machine wouldn't answer. I was climbing the walls! When he returned, he explained that his cleaning lady had accidentally turned it off.

- anything that keeps you from conveying information to the person you're trying to reach in a TIMELY fashion.

I realize that the good Lord was not generous to me in certain areas. He did not give me very much patience, I'm afraid, so I have a rough time when I can't at least leave a message for someone. These days there are a lot more people like me because of technology. The existence of all the cool technology that makes all of us always reachable is a double-edged sword. It has generated a lot of impatience, and a lot of frustration, often at the same time. As I always say, I have a love-hate relationship with my pager. I love it because people can always reach me. I hate it because people can always reach me.

People today expect to be able to reach everyone RIGHT NOW. At least, they want to be able to leave a message. When they call a business, they want the phone answered professionally, either by a voice mail system or by a live human being who knows how to take a message. If they call what is ostensibly a business, and get someone's roommate, who can't find a pencil, or someone's mother, who says "just a minute," then screams and hollers "it's for you!" they are not going to be prepared to place their trust in the person who comes to the phone, assuming someone does eventually.

Another thing that people have very little patience with today, a busy signal. In fact, many of us are shocked to hear one, in this age of voice mail. (For those of you who don't know what it is, a "busy signal" is a series of tones that means that someone is using the phone. This reminds me of the time I said, on the air, that I sound like "a broken record," then realized mid-sentence that at least a sizable minority of people in the audience, those born after 1980 or so, didn't know what that meant.) It's unbelievably annoying to be trying to give someone information, often that they themselves have requested, and hear that pulsing "beep-beep" on the other end of the line. With voice mail, that won't happen. If you're talking on the phone, incoming calls will go to your voice mail, and you can call them back. Potential clients won't be lost because of their irritation and frustration over not being able to reach you. Prospects who have a hard time reaching you will be thinking "what if I need to reach her after I've hired her?"

Thanks to the tremendous technological advances of recent years, voice mail systems are very affordable. Do yourself a favor and set one up. Otherwise, you'll never even know how many potential clients you're losing, not to mention how many other people you are annoying the hell out of.

Principle #15: Set up a professional communication system.

 Have you ever heard of HMB?

Remember that all personal trainers are teachers. All good teachers are lifelong learners. They have to be.

Have you ever learned a new word and suddenly you see it everywhere? That's what will happen with your clients when it comes to all the health and fitness news that they used to ignore. Not only will they start reading these articles, they will start highlighting them with a yellow highlighter, and then calling you up to ask you questions about them.

Fortunately, you will be one step ahead of them, provided, of course, that you keep reading. You'll have a few things going for you. If you subscribe to professional journals and magazines, you will be getting information first-hand. Most of the information that laypeople get in the popular press is, if not riddled with inaccuracies, simplified to the point of meaninglessness, especially if they get most of their information from television. Three minutes is an *extremely* long time on TV, so is it really possible for scientific information to get any serious treatment? "Is it true that cheeseburgers help you avoid getting cancer?" your client might ask, after seeing the latest TV expose. You get the idea.

Another problem with media reports that works to your advantage is that, for the sake of ratings, media outlets tend to sensationalize everything. Recently I got a press release from a PR flack who was trying to get a couple of her clients on my radio program. One was a so-called "Digestive Health Specialist" (people can be so creative about these made-up credentials, can't they?) who wanted to talk about colonics and other distasteful and, in my opinion unnecessary, procedures. Right into the circular file. The other one, though, a doctor who wanted to talk about essential fatty acids, was a definite maybe, provided he could lose the sensational approach reflected in the press release. "LOW FAT CONSPIRACY!!" the headline screamed. Good grief—would it be so bad for once to have a rational conversation about health? So many of these media weasels love the negative, the sensational and the intellectually-lazy. That works in your favor.

Finally, if you've got the right sort of relationship with your client, he will trust you much more than what he reads in the newspaper or hears on TV. Let's hear that you have at least that much more credibility.

The key to this principle is to remember that your client views you as an authority. Make sure you are aware of everything about health and fitness that is being reported in the popular media, and then some.

> **Principle #16: Read, read, read, and make sure you read the right stuff.**

 Tenzing Norgay is your new hero.

After a recent book signing, I was chatting with the store's manager and complimenting him on the attractive displays in the store. One such display was about outdoor adventure, and included the wonderful book, *Into Thin Air* by Jon Krakauer. The book tells the story of a disastrous expedition up Mount Everest. By way of background, Krakauer tells the story of the first documented successful expedition up Everest, that of Sir Edmund Hillary. On May 29, 1953, he became one of the first of two individuals ever to reach the summit of Mount Everest. I say "two" because Hillary was accompanied by his Sherpa, Tenzing Norgay, and neither man would say who reached the summit first. Both men always said they reached the summit together or, "We climbed as a team," neither one willing to accept credit, but both knowing that without the other, neither would have made it.

Their achievement highlighted the indispensable contribution of Sherpas in Everest expeditions. Commentators have noted that the Sherpas are not only extremely talented climbers, but seem to possess a unique attitude that enables them to perform their tasks not only with competence, but also with alacrity. (That's one of my favorite words. It means "cheerful enthusiasm.") The Sherpas performed with alacrity even in the severe conditions of Everest. Some have suggested that the reason may be the way that they view the mountain, and therefore their work. To the Sherpas, the mountain is a spiritual entity, and therefore their work is not a job, but a calling. Though originally employed as porters and assistants to haul the gear up the mountain, their burning determination and their indomitable spirit so impressed everyone who employed them that they became respected full partners, sharing in the shining moment on the top of the world.

I think that good personal trainers are like Sherpas. They must be strong. They must be reliable. They must be determined. And, like Sherpas, they must be attracted to the challenge and achievement of their job. The pay is good, but they aren't just in it for the money. They delight in being in the fortunate position of making money doing something they really love. Like Sherpas, though, personal trainers cannot do the long hard climb for their clients. We can only guide and support them. When the client reaches the summit of his personal fitness goal, he should be able to truly say to you, "I couldn't do it without you, but you can't do it for me." If you think of the trust and responsibility that is reflected in the work of Sherpas, and the respect they inspire in those they support, you'll have a good start in thinking of the way you should think of yourself as a personal trainer in a position of trust and responsibility.

Principle #17: Think of yourself as a Sherpa.

 Tomorrow belongs to those who have vision today.

OK, you've gotten the fact that it's not about you, but be honest, haven't you ever wanted to be inside someone's head to have them hear your encouraging voice when you're not there, to have them hear you reminding them of the different form points that they need to remember when they do an exercise? Of course you have. We all have. But there's being inside someone's head, and there's being inside someone's head. For example, the last time I heard "Muskrat Love"—don't ask me how that happened, because like any other major trauma, I've blocked it out—it kept playing inside my head for what seemed like several days, in an annoying, Chinese-water-torture sort of way. No, you want to be there like their memory of a beautiful spring day. The mere thought of you should inspire an endorphin surge. How can you do that? How can you occupy that special place in your client's head?

I mentioned that I have a radio show, but what you may not have thought of is that we all have a radio station playing in our heads all the time, WIIFM. WIIFM: What's In It For Me. We all pay more attention to information that we believe will affect our lives. Obvious, right? So the best way to achieve the goal of being inside your client's head even when you're not around, is to start out with agreed-upon objectives that you both buy into from the beginning. Some trainers seem to come up with objectives using the 3rd-person invisible method: the client is almost like a prop, and the objectives are like a bunch of bullet points in some boring business meeting agenda. These trainers may as well be talking to themselves, for all that they are engaging their clients in the process. Eventually, they will be talking to themselves because their clients <u>will</u> have moved on.

Clients typically begin with a lot of enthusiasm, and it's up to you to use that enthusiasm and to crystallize it into a shared vision of success. Enthusiasm is contagious, and it's your job to be a carrier.

It's also your job to keep reminding your client of his fitness dream and making it seem not only tangible, but achievable. Help him see it, feel it, smell it and taste it, then remind him that he can have it if he refuses to give up.

Vision means that your client learns not only the "how" when it comes to exercise, but also he learns the "why." Getting in shape is no different from any other important endeavor: the difficulty and the drudgery can easily overwhelm initial enthusiasm and obscure the pot of gold at the end of the rainbow. Vision is the eyes on the prize, it's the pot of gold at the end of the rainbow, the shining moment at the top of the world. It's the answer to that one question that is the secret to motivation, not only in exercise, but in every area of life: "What's the point?"

Principle #18: Be a visionary.

 Know your limits.

What is the ultimate tragedy? I think that while there is room for disagreement on this one—for instance, I think I could make a good case for my beloved Chicago Cubs—but I think that the ultimate tragedy is one thing that happens way too often: giving up. So I often think, as I look around, "Isn't it sad to look around and see so many people who still have so much to contribute to society and to themselves throwing in the towel at a really young age? They tell themselves that they're too old, too fat or too out of shape (or all three) to do the things that they'd like to do, the things that they could do to enrich their own lives and the lives of others. I think it was this tragic waste that first attracted me to personal training. As personal trainers, we have the power to help people reverse that way of thinking and overcome a lot of these self-imposed and, frankly, artificial limitations.

We must not conclude, though, that because we have the ability to point out how much control people have over their own health, that we have more control than they do themselves. One of our jobs as personal trainers is to teach them that they, *not we, not doctors, not anyone else*, hold the key to their own future health. Much like the Sherpa, we can help guide them up the mountain, point out hazards, give them a boost when they need it but, ultimately, they are in charge of their own health.

Some personal trainers, those for whom their sessions are their own personal ego-fest, seem to fear that if they explain to clients that clients are ultimately in charge, somehow that diminishes their authority and their power. But, remember, we're not involved in this profession to exercise power over people, or to have our egos stroked. We're in this profession to transform people's lives for the better. *It's not about you. It's about them.*

Repeating: No personal trainer, no guru, and no physician, has as much control over the short and long term health of any person as that person himself.

One of your most important jobs, and sometimes one of your biggest challenges, will be to get your clients to accept that reality because, while it is an extremely empowering statement, with power comes responsibility. Many times people want to avoid thinking about the fact that they really are in charge. They don't want that power because they don't want the responsibility. They'd much rather be able to say "fix me" to their trainer or in a worse case, their doctor. So one of your jobs will be to get them to not only accept, but to embrace, that responsibility without fear and with a certain amount of satisfaction and pride, knowing that they are exercising pro-active control over their own health.

The payoff is enormous. It's amazing what happens once people believe that they are in control of their own health, how that sense of power spills over into every area of their lives. You will see people make amazing strides forward, accomplishing things that they never knew that they could accomplish.

Ordinary people can do extraordinary things when you help them recognize the power that they've had all along.

> **Principle #19: Recognize that no one can change anyone else's behavior.**

 CPT? CPFT? XYZ?

My father told me that there were two kinds of people: those who do the work and those who take the credit. He said I should aim to be in the first group because there's less competition there. In our profession, that's sadly true: there are those who do the hard work of getting an education and mastering the knowledge we need to genuinely benefit our clients and those who I would call "posers," who want credit for being knowledgeable professionals without doing the work to deserve it. Their willing accomplices in destroying the effectiveness and reputation of our profession are club owners who view hiring the educationally-handicapped as a way to beef up their bottom lines. The public is the ultimate victim.

Do all of us a favor, if:

(1) you don't know anything other than what you read in one of those body-building magazines,

(2) you're certified by an agency that advertises on matchbook covers, whose sole criteria for certification is the ability to write a negotiable check, or

(3) you're just a good-looking bod who likes to work out and hang out in the gym

…please don't unleash yourself on an unsuspecting public. The world doesn't need one more dumb musclehead masquerading as a personal trainer.

Of course, today's dumb musclehead could be tomorrow's graduate. I'm not saying that if you don't have your degree TO-DAY, you can never join the club. The fact that you are reading this book shows that you want to be one of the top performers in our profession. I'm just saying this: just as the pre-med student doesn't do open-heart surgery, until you have a clue, as in some background, what you're doing might look like personal training, but it won't be very personal and the only one getting trained will be you. Clients shouldn't be guinea pigs for our on-the-job training.

Now, that that's out of the way, I hope you know that if you don't have any qualifications that allow you to legitimately put initials after your name, doing so just calls attention to this fact. It's like putting lots of makeup on a gigantic zit. You may think it covers it up, but it actually just highlights it like a big headlight. Do yourself a favor. If you want initials after your name, get an education.

Principle #20: Realize that attempting to inflate your qualifications makes you look bad.

 Legal Basic #1.

Earlier I mentioned the film "King of Comedy." In another scene, a group of guys are in a room, and someone says to one of them "So who are you?" He replies "I'm the lawyer. I'm the one who sues." I think that's the real reason that people hate lawyers: because they fear being sued.

Many personal trainers I've spoken to—students in my classes, and personal trainers I've been lucky enough to meet and talk to—seem first shocked and then terrified at the thought that they could be sued. Maybe you're feeling a little hinky right now. You need to relax. The fear of being sued is a bit like the fear of monster in your closet that you had when you were a child: the best way to get over it is to shine the light of truth on it, and to understand what is and isn't there.

Being a recovering lawyer-turned-personal-trainer has given me a unique perspective that has advantages and disadvantages. The disadvantage was that when I first got into the fitness field, I saw potential lawsuits EVERYWHERE. In fact, I still do. The advantage is that I realize that these are POTENTIAL problems.

A wise person once said that fear, F-E-A-R, is "False Expectations Appearing Real." And there's a lot of truth in that. What is understood is not feared, but handled. And that's what we're going to do: first by gaining an understanding of the legal basics, then by learning some practical tips and suggestions to help you stay on the right side of the law and finally, I will tell you the best protection you have against lawsuits.

We all know that there has been an explosion in medical malpractice cases over the last 25 years. I have a theory about that, which has nothing to do with greedy personal injury lawyers, which I'll revisit later. First I want to tell you about a conversation I had a with a client, who happens to be a physician. He somehow has managed to get himself into the unfortunate position of being in charge of cost containment, and no, he doesn't hold it against me that I call him an "HMO nazi." Recently he was lamenting the fact that he was constantly having to plead with his colleagues to stop giving patients so many— as he put it, "unnecessary tests." He said that whenever he asked why a doctor felt the need to give someone so many tests, the doctor would reply, "I don't want to get sued." I told him that he should say this: "Since anyone can sue anyone anytime, we can't let that affect our medical judgment. After all, I could sue you for divorce—and he was saying this to a male colleague—and until you went in to court and got it dismissed, you'd be "sued." It's stupid to base our patient care decisions on that." And it's true.

Recently the *Wall Street Journal* featured a story about a guy who found a great way to make a living. He was an ex-stockbroker who has figured out that by threatening to sue major corporations, he could extort $2000-$3000 out of them for the price of a stamp. Here's how it works: he sends them a letter, alleging that he, a shareholder of the company, was financially damaged by the board of directors' decisions. The company realizes that it would cost more than the two or three thousand he wants to hire a lawyer to get a case dismissed, so they just pay him off. It didn't matter that in most cases, *HE NEVER EVEN OWNED THE STOCK.* They didn't even check. It also didn't matter that he made only about $30,000 a year doing this. He doesn't need much money, since *HE'S IN PRISON.* There's a guy who gives new meaning to the term "jailhouse lawyer!"

Once you realize that anyone can sue anyone for anything anytime, it's a lot less scary, isn't it?

Principle #21: Don't let the fear of being sued paralyze you since anyone can sue anyone for anything.

 Legal Basic #2

For some reason, most people believe that waivers aren't worth the paper they're written on, but that's not true, if you do it right.

Here's the kind of waivers that courts uphold:

• *Clear and unambiguous*

This is no time to pussy-foot around. Let this be the first time that you hear this question, but it definitely won't be the last. This is a question that should always be in the back of your mind when it comes to working with clients "What's the worst thing that could happen?" Whatever the answer is, you need to say that *EXPLICITLY* in your waiver. My waiver form specifically mentions the risk of death during exercise. Have any clients ever died during a workout? No, but we all know that astounding and unexpected things can happen during exercise.

One day an employee of mine, a personal trainer, and I decided to try a spinning class at our club. Her husband, a lean, fit, non-smoking 35-year-old, decided to join us. We had a great time and all was well. About three weeks later, while running at the track, he collapsed in cardiac arrest. It was only then that doctors diagnosed a congenital heart defect. So bad things can happen when you least expect it, and your waiver needs to mention them.

• *Explicit*

You need to be explicit not only in describing the risks but also what activities you intend to cover with the waiver. If you're going to be doing fitness testing in addition to work-outs, be sure to cover that. If you're working out in the client's home, make sure you provide for the risks inherent in using equipment that you don't maintain or control. If you think of it, JUST SAY IT!

• *Consistent with State Law*

The law in this area is constantly changing. Not only that, but it varies state-by-state. Some state courts have defined "magic words" that you need to use to protect yourself. It's not your job to know those words. That's your attorney's job. Have your waiver form prepared by a qualified lawyer who knows your state's law and things should be just fine.

• *Knowing*

In addition to being clear, explicit and consistent with state law, a waiver is more likely to protect you if it is what lawyers would call a "knowing" waiver; that is, you don't want anyone to be able to say that it was signed without having first been read and under-stood, or that there was any pressure to sign it. I suggest that you send the waiver form to your new client well in advance of your first session, with a note telling him it is an important legal document that he might want to have reviewed by his attorney. Clients may not do this, but you want to offer the opportunity. If you send it to him in advance, no one can suggest that you were there pressuring him to sign it or that time pressure kept him from reading it.

Principle #22: Waivers will protect you, if you do them right.

 Legal Basic #3

Lawyers understand that there are four elements to a personal injury lawsuit:

- Duty
- Breach
- Causation
- Damages

In order for anyone to collect money from you (or your insurance company), he needs to prove that you were legally responsible to him in some way. That one's a no-brainer: personal trainers have a duty to provide supervision and instruction to their clients. Breach? That's the claim—that you didn't provide the appropriate supervision and instruction. The way lawyers would say it was that you didn't provide the supervision and instruction that a "reasonable and prudent personal trainer" would provide. The element of causation will be there if it can be proved that it was your fault, and not his or someone else's. So then we're left with damages: how much money did your mistake cost him? Lost wages, for example. Or loss of his ability to be a functioning husband and father. Whatever the lawyers can dream up.

OK. Now what if I slander you? I say that you had an affair with Bill Clinton along the lines of Monica Lewinsky, which is not true. As a result you get a six-figure book deal and your own talk show? Did I slander you? Yes. Can you sue me? Yes. Were you damaged? Maybe, but you'll have a hard time proving damages.

Always remember when people threaten to sue, they need to prove that they got hurt. Otherwise, they have no case. A lawsuit without damages is not a hammer: it's a squirt gun, annoying, but not dangerous.

Principle #23: A lawsuit without damages is not a hammer; it's a squirt gun.

The most important question you can ask during a workout

The number one rule in working with clients: never, never release your hold on a dumbbell or any piece of equipment without asking your client, "Do you have it?", and making sure that he has responded, "Yes.' Explain this to your clients. Explain that until they tell you that they have custody and control of that weight, you are not going to let go even if you have to stand there for five minutes. Sometimes it turns into a little bit of a joke. I had a client say to me recently, "Can't we just have that 'I have it' rule apply to dumbbells that weigh more than fifteen pounds?" The answer is, "No, of course not." How much damage could a three pound weight dropped from three feet onto a client's face cause? And remember, that's the burning question.

Here's another demonstration of how one simple question can save your client months of chronic pain and you lots of aggravation. As you probably know, the most vulnerable position for the shoulder is abduction and external rotation, for example during the pec dec exercise, with the forearms pressed against the machine's pads. A client of mine

---

sustained a chronic shoulder injury when he lost control of one of the pads on the pec dec, and it's easy to see why. Without complete custody and control of the weight stack, his upper arm snapped back, driving the head of his humerus bone back and up into what can only be euphemistically called an extreme mechanical disadvantage—OUCH! How could this happen to one of my clients? I wasn't with him at the time, and he just got distracted. Clients can sometimes get distracted, but it's your job to make sure you stay focused. If a client is chatting away as you begin an exercise, take a time out from the banter, and ask the one all-important question: do you have it? A few seconds of focus here can save months of trouble later.

> *Principle #24: NEVER let go of a piece of equipment that you hand to a client without asking, "Do you have it?"*

 #25   *Not because you want a cooler dumped on your head.*

In her very interesting, and occasionally frightening book, *Little Girls in Pretty Boxes*, Joan Ryan notes "the mythic image of coaches as physical and spiritual alchemists," that is very much a part of American culture. Consider the Hollywood images of coaches. From Pat O'Brien in "Knute Rockne, All-American" to Pat Morita in "The Karate Kid," and even Tom Hanks in " A League of Their Own," the template is as follows: surly and stingy with a compliment, but loyal to the end to their guys. Tough love personified, but more. Tough love and the ability to take some sorry wretch or wretches and transform them through the power of his personality, knowledge and sheer will into champions. Note the word "transform." That's what coaches can do. At least that's what they can do in the movies.

Like everything we see in the movies, you've got to take this image of coaches with at least a grain (sometimes a whole barge) of salt. (You don't really think that most of the people who own independent bookstores look like Meg Ryan and Hugh Grant, do you?) The kernel of truth that keeps the whole thing from being science fiction is this: a good coach can help a person find the ability inside themselves that was there all along. He can help his coachee be the best he can be, which we all know can sometimes be hard to do on our own. That's what you're going for here: trying to help your clients find the best in themselves.

To be your best, as you know, you sometimes have to look at yourself in a deep, dark truthful mirror, seeing yourself, warts and all. A good coach serves that capacity for his coachees, knowing that while in the short term he may have to help them face painful realities, in the long term the result will be a reflection that will delight them both.

The word "coach" is an acronym for the things you want to accomplish.

Communication

A client recently told me an amusing story about an attempt to schedule a meeting at his office. He thought the meeting was at 1 PM, but everyone else had a different idea of the correct time. Ironic isn't it: the subject of the meeting was supposed to be communication.

Remember that high-achievers tend to be stoic, and "you can observe a lot by watching." Our clients tend to be high-achievers, and they may not always tell you everything verbally. Learn to understand non-verbal communication.

Opening Doors

A trainer opens the door to better health and fitness, but a coach opens the door to the best person your client can be, as in:

- the door to overcoming fear
- the door to being in the present moment
- the door to letting go of things you can't control

But remember. . . you can open the door, you can't carry him over the threshold (refer to Principle # 17).

Accountability

Margaret Mead, the noted anthropologist, said that the oldest human need is to have someone wonder why you haven't come home at night. It is deep in human nature to want others to care about us. Your clients don't want to let you down.

Challenge

Setting goals for your client helps motivate him during times when he is in a motivational slump.

Health

Your most important goal for all of your clients should be long-term health and lifelong commitment to healthy lifestyle. Granted, they may come to you looking for that buff bod they saw in a television commercial, but like true love, which often starts with a zap of electricity and eventually develops into something deeper, most clients will come to the realization that what they're really looking for is more than skin-deep.

Principle #25: Strive to be a coach, not a trainer.

#26   *You're some body, (but fortunately, that's not all.)*

Some of my clients consider it a paradox for a "fitness person" to say what I'm about to say, but I'm constantly reminding them "you are not your body. It's just the house you live in." Does that sound strange to you, too? It shouldn't. I think that one of the reasons we have so many sedentary people, despite the constant drumbeat pounding away for the last ten years that everyone should exercise, the Surgeon General says, "blah, blah, blah," is the hard-body mentality. While I know that the corporate geniuses running certain large health club chains think that their television commercials featuring gyrating, lycra-clad muscle babes and stud muffins are beyond fabulous, I happen to know that to many people they are an intimidating turn-off. The sad reality is that even the people in these ads don't look this way most of the time (and the afore-mentioned corporate geniuses almost NEVER do, but that's another story), so what is really the point? To promote unrealistic, and for almost everyone other than full-time bodybuilders and professional fitness models, unattainable body images as the "ideal?"

I have a different philosophy, one that I hope you share. I think we should be encouraging people to want to develop strong and healthy bodies so that they will be able to use them to express the aspects of their personalities that make them unique: their intelligence, their senses of humor, and their creativity. Not only that, but to be able to express these things at their fullest for their entire lives, not just the first half or two-thirds. No one should spend the last third of his or her life sitting in a chair he has trouble getting out of. The body is the most amazing instrument any of us will ever possess, but it is just that, a tool that we use to interface with the world, not an end in itself.

A photographer I know once told me about a very enjoyable shoot he did with an 85-year-old woman. She told him that the most amazing thing about living to her advanced age was discovering that aging happened on the outside. On the inside, she still felt as if she were 25. Exactly.

> **Principle #26: The body is just the house the soul and spirit live in.**

 #27   *It's ok, Stubby, just put your feet up here on this bench.*

Have you heard about the doctor who went to heaven? Being a doctor, he was used to getting up to the front of the line, and this was no exception. He marched up to the head of the line and interrupted St. Peter mid-sentence with another new inductee. "Excuse me," he said, barely concealing his impatience. "I'm a physician, and I've just arrived, so I'd like to get to my room." One of the angels, noting St. Peter's irritation at the chuztpah of this guy, explained "I'm sorry, but you'll have to wait your turn like everyone else." So, the doc stomped angrily back to the end of the extremely long queue. As he stood there, fuming, he saw another doctor wearing a lab coat and stethoscope around his neck walk confidently to the front of the line. He said a few words to the angel and the gates opened immediately. Now our doctor-hero was really steamed. He stormed back up front and demanded to know why the other doctor could get in immediately when he couldn't. "Oh," the angel explained calmly. "That was God. Sometimes he likes to play doctor."

Yes, doctors can sometimes be know-it-alls. So can you imagine how exciting it is to have a doctor actually tell you that you taught him something? That happened to me once. All because I understand that each of us has different individual biomechanics. My doctor client was doing an incline bench press from time-to-time. He complained of back pain, especially immediately afterwards. I asked him to demonstrate the incline bench press for me. When he did, the problem was clear. His leg length and the height of the bench's seat forced him to reach a little to keep his feet on the ground. Instead of having them squarely planted and flat on the floor, he had them in tippy-toe position. Rather than his knees being at a comfortable 90-degrees, they were at a wavering 120 degrees or so. Not good. Looking around for something I could use as a footrest, I finally settled on a large dumbbell and placed it at the foot of the bench. I instructed him to sit back down on the incline bench and to put his feet on it. "How does that feel?" I asked. "Amazing," he said. "I'm cured!" He got a small footrest that he uses, and never felt the pain again. Placing a footrest at the base of an incline bench is one of the best things you can do to take stress off the low back. If you do it, you will delight and amaze most clients, especially those who have worked with other trainers who don't have a clue.

The take-home message here is that we all have individual biomechanics due to our distinctive body types. Some of us have long legs and short torsos. Others are the opposite. You need to pay attention to that. When you do, you will learn some very important and useful things. For example, you'll discover that certain machines are never going to work for certain people, and in those cases, you'll switch to free weight exercises to work certain body parts. You'll discover that your client can keep his back flatter during a dumbbell row on a higher (or lower, as the case may be) bench. One size fits all may work with those big gigantic nightshirts, but it doesn't work with exercise.

Principle #27: Recognize that because each of us has individual biomechanics, workouts should be designed and conducted accordingly.

#28 ***Well, I'll be switched! Who'd a thunk it?***

You'll be amazed, I know I often am, how easy it is to pick up two dumbbells of different weights and not notice the difference, one's a twelve and one's a fifteen or one's a ten and one's a twelve. I know I was, the time early in my career, when I did exactly that. I felt particularly stupid when one of the muscleheads standing nearby and observing began to guffaw loudly and bellowed "Some great personal trainer! You can't even see when the dumbbells are different sizes!" My cringe-o-meter still goes off when I think of that, despite the years that have passed and despite the fact that my client thought it was funny.

So this kind of thing is not necessarily a disaster, but it can make you look a little bit foolish in front of your client and at least temporarily diminish your effectiveness. If you hand the dumbbells to your clients, which I recommend, be sure that you check and make sure they are both the same weight when you do that. I recommend that you hand clients their dumbbells because that gives you a chance to make sure the dumbbells aren't loose or in some way broken. A lot of times, as you know, when you pick up these dumbbells in gyms, they're about ready to fall apart, usually because some bean bag has dropped them from about five feet in the air.

Regardless of the reason, you don't want to hand your client a dangerous piece of equipment, so check and double check everything. Check and double check whether cables are on the track of a machine. Check whether they're frayed. Check whether the machine is sticking or not. If you adjust the position of a seat, press on it to make sure it's stable, then sit on it yourself. This is the reason it's desirable when you're teaching a client to use a piece of equipment to demonstrate it first. It gives you an opportunity to check and double check that piece of equipment.

Principle #28: Always double check everything, and then check it again.

 #29 ***Phrases to eliminate from your vocabulary, at least in your conversations with clients.***

Most people don't intend to be offensive or hurtful when they talk. I certainly know that you don't. With the rare exception of the extremely ill-tempered, most verbal hurts inflicted are inflicted inadvertently. Still, if you run over someone with your car by accident, they're still hurt, whether you intended that result or not.

In my experience, it's impossible to completely avoid hurting people's feelings 100% of the the time, even if you're careful. There are, however, certain words and phrases that are like verbal lighter fluid: they can incite bad feelings faster than a phone call from the IRS. Here are the phrases that definitely DON'T pay:

"I know what you're trying to say"

Now, think about that one. It's another way of saying "You're a bad communicator, maybe even a moron who can't translate his simplistic thoughts into words, but fortunately, I am smart enough for both of us and I can figure it out." I know that some people at times speak as if English is their second language, even if it isn't, but that's no excuse for saying this obnoxious phrase. A better way of conveying the same thing is to back in with a question, as in "Do you mean _____?" and fill in the blank with what you think they mean. This way your client can clarify his original intent and you don't look like a rude oaf.

"Hang on"

Excuse me? Maybe I don't want to hang on! That's my first reaction when I am unfortunate enough to be on the receiving end of that phrase. That's true even when I've initiated the call and really want to speak to the person at the other end of the phone. Why is this so bad? Because it says "Oh, you insignificant little person, you have all the time in the world, obviously, so there's not doubt that you can wait while I deal with more important matters than you. I don't have to ask you whether you can wait. That's a given." It's not, though, and even if it is, assuming it is rude! Better way to say the same thing: "I'm sorry, but could I possibly ask you to hold for just a minute?" Of course, if it's going to be more than a minute, tell the caller so, and ask whether he'd prefer to hold or to be called back. Show respect for other people's time.

"No," as the first word in a sentence

"But, Ter, but Ter," I can just hear you guys, "it's an honest answer." So? As I always used to tell my clients when I was practicing law, some things are better left unsaid (and DEFINITELY unwritten, but that's another story.) I'm not saying that you have to be like the character in the play "Oklahoma," the girl who couldn't say no. As much as you'd like to, and as accommodating as I know you try to be, it won't always be possible for you to say yes to every request. That's a given. The question isn't whether you have to say no or not. The question is how you say it. Starting a sentence with the word no is harsh. To the hearer, it's like being slapped up the side of the head with a two-by-four, or at least a wet washrag. Instead, try this one "I'm afraid I won't be able to change your appointment to Friday at 5 PM this week, but I'll definitely let you know right away if anything changes.

Is there any other time that might work almost as well?" This type of statement conveys concern and a desire to accommodate your client. "No, I can't make it Friday at 5 PM" says the same thing in substance, anyway, but without the concern and caring so essential to positive communication and good client relations.

A special note to you high-tech types: all of this goes double in e-mail.

Principle #29: Make your communication positive.

Busier than a one-armed paperhanger.

Once a client, who happens to be a physician, and I were working out together in the gym. We saw a guy with his left leg in a cast from his ankle up to his hip, hobbling around, dodging all of the obstacles that make gym floors the minefields that we know them to be. I felt sorry for the poor wretch because it was obvious that he was looking for something, anything he could do to experience the euphoria that a workout can bring. Workout withdrawal is the worst! Fortunately, as we explained, you don't have to sit idly by and atrophy when you have an injury, even one serious enough to require immobilization. To quote Teddy Roosevelt, 'do what you can with what you've got where you are'. In other words, research has shown that if the uninjured limb is trained, the injured leg will not atrophy as much.

The human brain is the most amazing object in creation, so it's no surprise that it contains this, as well as many other, amazing abilities.

Most of us know that people tend to be right- or left-dominant. Try it yourself, and you'll see that you are able to lift more weight with one limb or the other. Sometimes clients, and even trainers, are surprised because the side that they expect to be dominant, usually the right side in most people, won't be stronger. I think that that's because the dominant side will be tired out from doing most of the days' activities all day. When you explain this to clients, they get very interested in helping the other side catch up.

As a personal trainer trying to optimize the effectiveness of your client's programs, it's important to consider that they are bilateral creatures. When you design your clients' routines, make sure to have them do some exercises one leg and one arm at a time. Obviously, this will work best on single-joint movements like leg extensions, leg curls and dumbbell bicep curls, but consider being creative, at least with your more advanced clients. How about a single-leg leg press, for example? A lunge with a foot up on a bench? Not only will including these exercises make things more interesting, you will be training strength, as usual, as well as balance and functionality.

One client, knowing how enamored I am of this strategy, once asked me "Single or double?" as he approached the leg curl machine. "Wow, I replied. "If you can do that standing leg curl both legs at once, that will really be something!"

Principle #30: Do at least some resistance training one limb at a time.

 Those guys on ER get to do it every week, but you can't!

Your mother told you not to play doctor, and she was right! Since you have your client's best interests at heart, you don't want to exceed the limits of your expertise. For example, like most people who exercise, most clients are going to get aches and pains. More important, they are going to ask you what to do about their aches and pains. When they do, you need to make sure that you help them. Sometimes the best way to help someone is to convince him to get to the doctor STAT.

I'm not saying that you can't make general suggestions about simple things like sprains or tendonitis. For example, there's nothing wrong with saying something like "Of course, I'm not a doctor, but I know that when I get that sort of pain I go with the standard RICE (Rest, Ice, Compression and Elevation) routine. If it lasts more than a couple of days and doesn't seem to be improving, though, I suggest you consult your doctor." I would steer clear of recommending medications, even over-the-counter ones. I know that sounds overly cautious, but I don't think you can be too careful with this one.

Giving medical advice can get you in lots of trouble. Let's say your client has an injury, nothing major. On your advice, he takes some over-the-counter anti-inflammatories and keeps working out as usual. The thing doesn't improve, but he figures you know what you're talking about, so he still doesn't seek medical attention. By the time he finally does, the injury has progressed from something minor to something serious. Suddenly, he doesn't call you. Unfortunately, someone you don't know, does. Surprise: It's his lawyer!

Not only can you be sued, but in most states there is a crime on the books called "Unauthorized Practice of Medicine." In my state, Illinois, even representing yourself as a doctor in an attempt to confuse or defraud the public is a felony. Unless, of course, you're doing a guest appearance on ER.

Principle #31: Practice good personal training, not bad medicine.

#32   *If your client were a car, you would be. .*

Often when I give speeches, I compare our bodies with our cars. "If I approached you with a beaker full of liquid of unknown origin, and told you that you should pour it into your gas tank, most of you would look at me as if I had grown another head, and say 'I don't think so!' and of course, you'd be absolutely right!" I go on to explain that it doesn't make sense, then, that we often eat things that come from God knows where and do God knows what!

I think the car analogy also works when it comes to your relationships with your clients. Consider the following ways that you are like components in your client as car:

Guidance System

Like one of those computer generated map systems, there you are, charting the course by helping your client set goals, both in the beginning and at every new level of progress, even if he doesn't want to ask for directions.

Steering Wheel

Sometimes clients get in a slump and they end up in the ditch, figuratively (at least I hope it's figuratively!) Sometimes they need help when they come to the fork in the road. During these times, your job is setting them straight and on the path to greatness.

Brake

A lot of us think that our job is to push our clients to go farther, faster and harder, balls to the wall, but sometimes your job is helping them understand when to back off. We get stronger, after all, not during training, but during recovery.

Mirror

Obstacles to progress might be in his blind spot, but you'll alert him to these dangers and pitfalls. In addition, like seeing his reflection in the mirror, by seeing himself through your eyes, he will unconsciously strive to be his best.

Principle #32: Use analogies your clients can understand to help them appreciate your role in their lives.

#33　　　*Two steps forward, one step back, but that's ok.*

Most of the people I work with drive themselves harder than a prison foreman supervising a chain gang. They are overachievers, and failure is not something they expect. In fact, it's barely in their vocabularies. They are goal-oriented, pro-active, and all those other buzzwords from the success self-help guru guys. They live the seven habits, the fifth discipline and the ten steps to empowerment. In short, they are people who expect results and usually get them. That's why sometimes it's so hard for them to understand why their progress in their exercise and weight control programs is not always up-up-up. You may understand that progress is not always in a linear progression, but you need to spend some time, especially in the beginning, explaining it to them.

Setbacks are inevitable. We all experience illnesses, injuries, business travel, family problems, and other challenging situations involving the propensity of life to slap us up the side of the head. When that happens, we need to take a step back and re-group. Sometimes this will mean settling for less intensity in our workout regimens. And, as Stuart Smalley might say, that's ok. After all, exercise is a lifetime activity, and over the course of 50 or 60 years, what's a couple of weeks, or even months?

One strategy to help clients keep setbacks in perspective is to teach them to focus not on the outcomes, but on the process itself. Encourage him to stop worrying about the results from his program next week or next month, as in "when will I be down to 18% body fat?," and instead to think about how he feels during and after a workout. Appreciating how good it feels to breathe deeply and feel his blood pumping, and then basking in the sense of accomplishment of a workout well-done is one of the greatest motivators of all.

> **Principle #33: Anticipate setbacks, and help your clients prepare for them.**

 #34　　　*I have no trouble taking you seriously, but I think you need to put some pants on.*

I've always had this theory of career choice. You should choose your career by picking something that allows you to wear the clothes in which you feel most comfortable. Hey, you're thinking, then personal training must be the job for me. I love wearing baggy sweats one day and skin-tight lycra the next. I love being able to wear just about any old thing I like. Read on, Sparky, for more about that wearing what you want thing. (Short answer: you're wrong.) I agree, though, it's nice to be liberated from the old suit-and-tie or nylons-and-pumps thing, which is why I was so surprised when I visited a small work-out facility operated by a proponent of the "SuperSlow" method of resistance training—what am I saying, he was a zealot. He called my radio program to talk about it and he wanted me to come to his place to put me through my paces. "I'm game," I joked, "but don't shoot me." The workout was interesting and tough, but the thing I remember most was that Mr. SuperSlow wore a suit and tie when he took me through it. When I first saw him, I commented on this unusual attire for a personal trainer. He explained that he believed we should dress like other health professionals, say doctors. As we went through the workout, I realized there was no reason for him not to wear a suit and tie. After all, he was only resetting the seats on machines and moving the pins on the stacks.

While I don't share his philosophy entirely (I mean, I don't see myself in nylons and pumps taking a client through a tough set of squats), I think he has a point. Simply because we are lucky enough to work in a profession like fitness where we don't have to wear stifling business attire, does that mean we should walk around dressed like we barely escaped a house fire, wearing ripped or even stained, or even worse, dirty clothes? I don't think so, but I've seen some personal trainers who look a tad casual. OK, forget the charitable euphemism—they look like rag pickers! You may say, quite accurate, that it shouldn't make any difference. You're being hired for your professional advice and judgment, and it shouldn't matter what you wear, as long as it's clean. That reminds me of people who complain that they have no social life, but refuse to make any effort at their appearance. They're right: people shouldn't be so superficial. They're so right that they can spend every Saturday night home along thinking about it because, right or not, it's reality.

If you want to be respected as a professional, you can run around like a lycra-clad bimbo or a steroid-mad musclehead. Those hardbody-displaying outfits that look great on you may either intimidate or annoy your client (or his wife). You shouldn't take the chance. Instead, opt for conservative workout apparel, like warmups or even tights with a baggy shirt over it. Your credibility will be enhanced, and you won't have to keep your stomach sucked in so hard.

Principle #34: Dress like a professional.

#35   ***It's the politeness of kings, after all.***

When I arrived at her house, I found my long-time client agitated. When she saw me, she had that look that your mom used to get when you wandered off at the beach: she's thrilled to see you, and she wants to smack you. What was the cause of this consternation? I was supposed to be there at 7:30 am, and it was 7:36!

If you knew me as well as she does, you'd be worried, too, You see, I pride myself on being on time for appointments. I see it as a respect issue. Now, anyone can have an emergency, but if you're consistently late, it's as if you're saying "my time is worth more than yours, so you can just wait." You may have never thought of it that way before, unless, of course, someone has kept you waiting. When you're the one waiting, maybe even worrying, minutes seem like hours. You don't know what to do—should you call? Open up your briefcase and do some work? But what if you do and then suddenly just as you get situated, the bonehead shows up! If you put yourself in the position of the "waitee," you'll get some appreciation for how annoying it is.

So being late is a way of "dissing" your client. That's the most important reason, in my opinion. There are also two others that you should consider:

- One reason that clients hire trainers is to help them fit their workouts in, to keep them on schedule. The last thing they need is another person to make them fall farther behind. They've already got their kids, spouses, co-workers and assorted timewasters to do that!

- Your time is your stock-in-trade, and if you treat it loosely, so will clients. Suddenly, they will get lots of cancellations and clients who show up late or inconsistently. What goes around, comes around, and what you treat seriously, they will treat seriously.

To avoid being late, I suggest that you familiarize yourself with the best, and also alternative routes for getting to every client destination. I think it's a good idea to drive to the place the day before just to get the lay of the land.

In addition, technology can really improve your customer service. If your life is anything like mine, you'll find yourself spending a large part of the day going from pillar to post, seeing clients, running errands, working out, and God knows what else. Every week will be different. If you find yourself between client appointments, you should probably use that time to take care of some of those errands, but that could put you in a situation where you are either going to be five minutes early or five minutes late. Digital phones were made for this situation! Call your client and see which one he prefers. In the unfortunate, and I hope extremely rare, case that you can't help being late, use the phone to let your client know you're on the way and suggest she start warming up. It's not your fault some imbecile decided to try to get his 12' semi under an 8' viaduct!

> ### Principle #35: Be punctual.

 #36   *Sometimes you're the windshield. Sometimes you're the bug.*

Do you ever have days when you don't feel like working out? Me, never? Oh, not much! Of course, I do, and I know you do, too. On those days, you are just dying to have someone beat you like a red-headed stepchild, right? If the answer is 'no,' then why do so many trainers assume that that's what clients want? "Because, Ter," I can hear you protesting, "that's why they hire us! To push them! To make them reach back in the country and get some more! To go heavy or go home!" You're right, but only some of the time.

This is such an individual thing. Understanding it and applying it effectively will challenge not only your coaching skills, but your interpersonal relationship skills. Recently one of my training partners suffered the horrific tragedy of having her husband die unexpectedly. It was very painful for those of us who are close to her. I can't imagine the pain she must have been enduring. The surprising thing was it seemed like most days working out helped, and it seemed like she wanted to really push it in the gym. I think it was a relief for her, an escape. That's the sort of stoic person she is. There are others, though, for whom the best thing would have been just some stretching and low-intensity cardio. Anything else would have been too difficult under the circumstances. Now, here's something important to understand, something key: I said that <u>most days</u> working out helped. There were other days when she just couldn't handle it, stoic or not.

Your clients are going to have good days and bad days. On some of the latter, they are going to be distracted and have a crummy workout. On some of the former, they will be ticked off and they will take out their anger on the weights. On those days, they will be stronger than you've ever seen them. Sometimes the same person will experience different reactions to the same stimulus. YIKES! This is really complicated! Fortunately, you're up to the challenge.

> ### Principle #36: Learn when to use the carrot and when to use the stick.

#37   *Quick—strip off those plates so I can pump out a few more!*

We've all seen the muscleheads in the gym. You know, the guys screaming at the tops of their lungs "It's all you, Man. Two more! C'mon, Man!" Ok, they're fun to watch. It's funny and everything, but don't emulate them, for goodness sake!

Especially this thing they do where they don't put collars on the bar! What's up with that? I know they think that the extra nanosecond it might take their spotter to take the collars off and remove a couple of plates during their cool "breakdown" set will destroy its intensity, but we know better. More likely, when the guy is doing the last rep, really reaching back for that one magical one, he'll push the bar up unevenly and all the plates on one side will go crashing to the floor, while the bar drops and smacks him the face. Maybe that would serve him right. Make sure you don't deserve to be smacked by making the same stupid mistake.

It may seem more time-efficient to skip the collars on bars and pins on seats, and all the little things that make equipment safer, but it's a big mistake. The risk of something going wrong, and the resulting negative impact if something does go wrong, greatly outweighs any perceived benefit.

> **Principle #37: Always use collars.**

 #38   *Of course I'd die if my husband ever found out.*

You will not believe some of the things your clients tell you. Really funny things. Really useful things. Really personal things. Once you get to that Level 3 relationship with your client, you are more than a coach and a trainer. You are a trusted confidant. Sometimes you're one of the few people that your clients believe they can talk to. Many of them are in positions of responsibility and are expected to be strong and stoic all day long. When you show up, they are bursting at the seams to unload on someone. I would love to tell you some of the things they've told me—talk about juicy reading—but then that's just the point, isn't it?

The point is that they'll tell you serious personal things, and it's up to you to keep those things private. As in you don't tell <u>anyone</u>. I have an advantage here over some of you. In my first career, as an attorney, keeping client confidences private is one of the rules to live by.

Nor do you talk about your clients and their problems in public, even if you don't use any names. I was so embarrassed one day in a gym locker room when I overheard someone who claimed to be a trainer and a "motivational speaker" (yeah, right) going on about all the "emotional problems" she helps her clients overcome. Oh, the burdens this genius must have to bear on behalf of all of these poor wretches lucky enough to have her in their lives! Stop me before I hurl! If any of her clients could have heard her condescending little rap, I think that they would have not only fired her immediately, but I'm sure that they would have felt personally betrayed and very hurt. The trainer-client relationship is about trust, and trust means respecting people's feelings and privacy, even when they aren't around.

Another point to consider about privacy is that things that you might not consider embarrassing or humiliating if they happened to you might be very embarrassing to your client. For example, a client might tell you about an ice cream binge involving several whole cartons in a single weekend. Your attitude might be (I would say quite correctly) "so what? we all screw up sometimes." In your client's eyes, though, this is a horrific personal failure and one that he'd rather not have the whole world know about. Always evaluate information from your client's point of view, not your own.

> ### Principle #38: Respect your client's privacy.

 ### You can't work in, Bitch! So get the !@#$% away from the squat rack!

The foregoing is a direct quote from a member of a gym where I had taken my client. The gym was a nice place, but, as you know, even in nice places, bad things can happen. Even worse, it was uttered mere inches away from my face with my horrified client watching, mouth agape. Here's what happened: My client and I were all psyched up for a good squat workout. We approached the rack, and asked the other members around if anyone was using the rack. "We haven't seen anyone," everyone agreed. Ok! As we began to prepare the bar by putting the plates on, we were startled by a shrill, ear-splitting sound that was vaguely human. Actually, it sounded like someone was getting sex change surgery with a corkscrew. We looked around to see a well-known steroid-guzzling freak charging toward us. (Well, the sex change appeared to be working, anyway.) "She" then uttered the afore-mentioned unforgettable phrases. What an eloquent and friendly greeting! Did I take her hideous, freakish face, scarred from way too many hours in the tanning bed, and slap it with the nearest dumbbell? I wanted to, but instead, I said nothing as I hustled my client away from there, then tried to make the best of a very frightening and disconcerting situation. I followed up with a certified letter to the gym's management, describing the incident and suggesting that they have a talk with her immediately.

The key to this principle is to put your ego aside and think of your client. In the short-term, the important thing is to get him away from any similar psychos that you are unfortunate enough to encounter immediately. There will be time to explain 'roid rage later, and you definitely should. Some clients have a really hard time even going into a gym in the first place. After something like this happens, they regress to the level of discomfort they had on the very first day.

In the long-term, assuming the incident occurs in a public gym or club, you should document the event in writing to management, preferably by certified letter. Be sure to keep a copy for your files.

The good news is that this sort of incident is extremely rare in my experience. I just want you to be able to handle it if you happen to be one of the "lucky" ones like me. (If I have to be the one who beats the odds, why couldn't I have won the lottery?)

Principle #39: Protect your client from gym freaks.

 Excuse me, but could I interrupt you for a second? I can't re-member what I'm supposed to do next.

Gyms can be fascinating places. There is so much going on that sometimes when I'm in the gym I get a sense of sensory overload. Between the pounding beat from the aerobics room, the clanging and banging in the free weight area and the ambient conversation, it's almost impossible to hear yourself think at times. It's easy, then, to get distracted.

Your clients are going to notice this right away. One of your challenges is keeping them focused on the specific exercise you're doing and the form that you're trying to teach him. And "challenge" is the right word, believe me. When you're trying to instruct a 50+ matron, who managed to set foot in the free weight room ONLY because she knew you'd be with her—"Maybe it won't be too scary if I'm not alone"—and the air is suddenly filled with the loud crash and the primal scream that sometimes accompanies the triumphant completion of a heavy set by one of the muscleheads, she's going to lose focus! You'll be lucky if she doesn't run out of the room like her sweats are on fire. OK, I'm exaggerating, but her eyes will probably get as big as saucers and she'll look to you to get things back on track. So, even though you might be distracted, too, you have to have the ability to almost immediately switch gears back to the matter at hand: your client.

Of course, it's not only those of you who work in clubs who have to worry about focus. There are a million distractions in people's homes, probably more than in the gym or health club. Don't find yourself fascinated by a story on TV, only to be jolted back to reality by hearing your client's pleading entreaty "Did you hear me?"

> **Principle #40: Focus your attention where it should be—on your client.**

 Does anybody really know what time it is?

One thing that I hope you're realizing about these principles is that they are all synergistic. If you do things right, you'll have a standing book of clients who are cult-like in their devotion to you. You won't be spending much, if anything, on marketing most of the time. You won't be scrambling to pay your bills or yourself. In other words, life will be good.

Good for you, and also for your lucky clients. Your relationships with them will all be Level 3 relationships (refer to principle # 9), so you'll understand exactly what they need from you and how to deliver it. Best of all, you will truly enjoy each other's company.

Sometimes I feel guilty keeping my clients past the time our sessions end because I'm so busy chatting them up about work, projects we're both working on, movies we've seen (or don't want to see because they look WAY too stupid). They never seem to mind, and I finally do leave, feeling grateful once again for the fact that I can not only do something I love to do, but also do it with such great people.

Not that you shouldn't be willing to spend an extra few minutes even with new clients, especially with new clients. They're the ones with lots of questions, right?

I can just hear some of you "But, Ter, but Ter, what about undervaluing and underpricing our services? If we stand around chit-chatting, aren't we giving away time, which, after all, is our stock and trade?" Ah, but remember, I was talking about pricing as a strategy to increase your practice at the beginning. What we're talking about here is the long-awaited and happy time after you've got all the clients you can provide your terrific service to. With this group, there's no place for clockwatching. In other words, if you don't think you have the time at the end of a session to answer a few questions, or if you don't think you have time to do a favor for a client on your time, you may have too many clients. Your goal should be to provide the very best in customer service to as many people as you can. Sadly, that may not be that many people, but that's why the few and the proud who are lucky enough to be your clients are willing to pay two or three times as much to you as they are to the trainers down at the club.

Principle #41: Don't be a clockwatcher.

 Dem, dere and dose.

No, that's not what I mean. I'm not expecting you to adopt your clients' regional accents, but you should try to adapt your manner of speaking to theirs. It's subtle, but we all have distinctive ways of phrasing things. Some of us speak formally. Even the use of the word "speak" instead of the word "talk" would be notable in certain circumstances.

It's not just choice of common words. Beware of technical jargon. One day I was with a client and she was doing a tricep exercise. The effectiveness of this exercise, like most tricep and bicep exercises, is dramatically improved by keeping the elbows in line with the shoulders, in other words, what you or I might call "internal rotation." As she proceeded through her set, I noticed, as is often the case as fatigue sets in, that she began to turn her elbows out, and I said "internally rotate, please." She looked at me blankly, like a puppy who wants to do as commanded, but who is clueless about how to please his master. "I mean 'elbows in,' " I said, quickly correcting myself. She smiled and immediately corrected her form. She wanted to do what I wanted her to do, but I had to say it in language she could understand. If your client is a physician, as several of mine have been, it's perfectly acceptable to use anatomical terms for body landmarks, but if you say 'scapula' to some of your clients, their going to think you're talking about a kitchen implement used to flip pancakes. For most people, 'shoulder blade' is a much better choice.

Principle #42: Gear your language to match your client's.

 As long as you're reading so much, anyway. . .

I have a client who says I'm the only person he's ever met who reads both *the National Enquirer* and the *Wall Street Journal*. He's right, although I hasten to point out that I have a subscription to the latter, and read the former while in line at the supermarket. I've got to have something to distract me from counting the number of items of the person in front of me in the (so-called) express lane and then doing a slow burn. One reason my clients know what I read is that they are quite likely to be beneficiaries of my informal clipping file. If I see something that might be of interest, out come my little clipping scissors.

It's just another way to let your clients know that you are thinking of them all the time, even when you're not with them. In itself, that's a good thing for a lot of reasons, some of them less significant than others. It keeps you in the front of his mind, which is good if he happens to be at a party and someone tells him how great he looks, then asks who his personal trainer is. In my opinion, that's a less significant reason. Going up the ladder of importance, consider how motivating it will be for your client to always have it in the back of your mind that you're always thinking of him. If you're always thinking of him, then in his mind, that means he's accountable to you. At least that seed has been planted, and that can't help but keep him more consistent.

I don't limit this little service to active clients alone. Sometimes a client will go on "independent study" for a while, for example, during a time when work is particularly stressful and they want the flexibility of working out any time of day. I'll give them homework to do, and we stay in touch by phone or e-mail. Sometimes you'll get a client who wants to work with you only so long as it takes to get familiar with exercises and equipment. You write a program and teach him how to do it with a view to checking in with him next quarter or thereabouts. Sending clippings of interest to these inactive clients is a great way to make sure they don't forget about you.

It's a little thing, that like so many other little things, can have a big impact.

Principle #43: If you see an article about an area that interests your client, send it to him.

 #44   *You say it's your birthday.*

I don't know how you feel about your birthday. Some people dread it. I, on the other hand, always look forward to mine. For one thing, it's the one time a year that I indulge in a gooey cake. And then there are all the presents. It's more than that, though. The real reason is that the passage of time is inevitable, and all things considered, I'd rather have a birthday than the alternative.

Clients appreciate it when you remember their birthdays, even if they aren't thrilled to be another year older. There's another reason to remember birthdays. They are a good opportunity to reiterate that the ultimate goal of all of this fitness stuff is, as one my favorite professors used to say, to die young at a very old age.

Of course, it's not only birthdays that you should note. I draw the line at the phony greeting card company-concocted holidays, but I think you should acknowledge genuinely significant events like children's graduations, baptisms, promotions and anything else that your client thinks is important. One of the first things I ever ordered on line was flowers to send to a client who had to put one of her beloved dogs to sleep. I made a big difference in how she felt, not only about the sad event, but about me as her coach and her friend.

Principle #44: Remember client occasions.

 I have just what you need. Of course, I just happen to sell it.

If I had a nickel for everyone who ever asked me to "represent" their line of supplements, I'd be richer than God. OK, I'm exaggerating, but not a month goes by when someone doesn't want to tell me how much I can help my clients, and more important, they always stress, how much money I can make, by selling supplements or some related product. One multi-level marketing bonehead actually knocked on the door of my home, hoping to drop in and chat about his cool products. I don't think so! I don't like it when my best friends in the world come over unannounced, so obviously this dude and I were not meant to be fast friends. Nor were we going to be business partners in this lifetime.

I understand the reason that so many people in our profession feel the need to sell vitamins, magnets, and related fitness products. Until that human cloning thing is perfected, there is a limit to how many people you can see, and therefore how much money you can make, one-on-one. After all, as terrific as you are, you are only one person. I'm not going to tell you that you shouldn't sell supplements, weight loss products, magnets and whatever else you can think of to clients. I will tell you, though, that I never have and I never will.

Don't get me wrong. I have nothing against supplements. I take many myself. When clients ask me which ones, I'm more than happy to tell them and why. Then I recommend that they read as much as they can about the subject so that they can make an informed decision. I view anything else as a conflict of interest. I never want to be in the position of having my financial interest dictate, or even help me rationalize, recommending something to a client that might not be the best thing for him. I also think that people are so desperately engaged in the endless search for the elusive "magic pill" that it's a little unfair to exploit this desire.

On the other hand, trainers who disagree with me would say that if they really like a product and think it's the greatest thing since sliced bread, it would be a disservice NOT to tell their clients about it. And, of course, if they're going to tell them about it, why shouldn't they benefit, too? It's a win-win. Skeptics like me reply that we don't think it's a coincidence that whenever anyone approaches us to hawk a product, they always start out, "Believe me, I never had any desire to sell anything like this before. I always hated this stuff, until I found THIS product."

This is one that you need to decide for yourself. All I want you to do is to think about it first.

Principle #45: Avoid potential conflicts of interest.

 I'm from the Federal Government and I'm here to arrest you.

Probably one of the most damaging contributors to the reputation of personal trainers as a bunch of dumb muscleheads is the fact that many personal trainers ignore the simple conventions that govern other businesses. Just because you don't carry a briefcase, or don't wear a suit every day doesn't mean that you should be showing up at your sessions and collecting money from your clients like some kind of a street musician. Take the time to establish some invoicing procedures and other simple paperwork that will not only make you appear more professional to your clients, but will also reduce your risks of having any unpleasant encounters with government agencies like—dare I say it?—the IRS. Sadly, just because you wear lycra or sweats, doesn't mean that you, like every other small business, aren't subject to being set upon our friends at the IRS. But if you have some good bookkeeping procedures in place, that fact will be less likely to cause you to lose sleep at night.

A Case Where Fear May be Justified

If there's any group of people who are more despised than lawyers, it's probably those fine public servants at the IRS. Ask yourself: if an IRS agent and a lawyer were drowning, what would you do? Go to lunch or read the paper? Right. People hate and fear the IRS for good reason. Those three letters are enough to strike fear into the hearts of even the most honest taxpayer. When you consider three facts: (1) the ridiculous complexity of the tax laws (2) while recently Congress has been working on changing the burden of proof so that it is on the government and not the taxpayer, the IRS has always been the guilty-until-proven innocent branch of our government and (3)the agency's ability to collect not only back taxes, but also penalties and interest dating back to the date that they say you should have paid, it's no wonder.

Horror Stories

I'm not here to scare you, but if I were, I'd just tell you horror stories about IRS abuses. OK, maybe just one or two.

How about when the IRS claimed that a businessman owed back taxes and it threatened to seize the iron lung which kept his polio-stricken wife alive unless he paid up?

How about the police officer in Kansas City who made the mistake of giving a ticket to an IRS agent? He was "randomly" selected for an audit. After nothing could be found wrong with his taxes, the IRS continued to spy on and harass him for four months before finally admitting that he owed them nothing.

Stories like this are why few things in life can ruin your day like a letter with a return address reading "IRS," but by the time you've finished reading this, you'll be prepared to avoid unpleasant close encounters with the ever-popular guilty-until-proven innocent branch of our government.

Principle #46: Establish a professional bookkeeping system.

 #47   *You're crazy and I hate you. Not really.*

Once on the radio show, I told a story about a guy hitting on me in the gym. Maybe I'm not being fair to him. Maybe he was just trying to be friendly, but it sounded like a come-on. He heard me say to my (also female) training partner that "men and women are different." This is a statement that for my money comes as close as anything to indisputable, but he saw an opening anyway. He approached me and, in his suavest voice suggested "Maybe we're not so different. Maybe you've just met the wrong guys." I couldn't resist being my usual obnoxious self. I said "Trust me. I may have met lots of the wrong guys, but for many years I've been with the only guy who could stand me!" My husband is an amazing human being in many ways, but the relevant thing here is that I KNOW he's amazing. I know how hard I am to live with for more reasons that I can list here.

When I told this story to a male friend, he lamented the fact that his ex-girlfriend couldn't have this attitude. He commended me on my ability to see the male point of view. I told him that I guess it was easy for me. Not only am I in touch with my male side: it's a big part of my job.

And also of yours. It's called empathy, and if you haven't already done so, you need to check into it. So many of these principles are really about that: empathy, the ability to put yourself completely in the place of another and understand his feelings as you understand your own. In the case of your clients, that might mean, at times, that you need to put your own feelings and your own ego completely aside. That's very tough, but to be a good coach, you've got to be able to do it. For example, once I had a client who was under a tremendous amount of stress at work, and without going into alot of detail, let's just say that I inadvertently added to his stress by suggesting that he help me with something. When he told me that I had added to his burdens, I was mortified. I had made every effort to reduce his stress, and now I had made it worse! I apologized profusely and made a solemn vow to myself to try harder to make sure this never happened again. Several days later when we were talking, he remarked on this situation by telling me, half-jokingly, that I was "banned" from his workplace (as if my mortification over what happened hadn't caused me to impose my own "ban") because I am "crazy." (He explained that he meant that I'm so serious about my work that most people think I <u>look</u> crazy, but that didn't make it better in my eyes.) This feeble attempt at humor wounded me to my core—it still hurts a little as I write this—and the unfairness of it stung like a slap. It took a great deal of emotional control to put it behind me. When the stress at work died down, we dealt with it, and repaired not only our professional relationship, but our friendship.

The take-home message for you is that sometimes you need to forget your own feelings, sometimes so much so that you have to completely step outside yourself, and put yourself in your client's shoes, even when it hurts. It's not always easy, but it's essential if you're going to be your best.

Principle #47: Recognize the importance of empathy.

 Should I lift light weights for lots of reps, or heavy weights for low reps?

Periodization is the gradual cycling (allocation of specific time, whether days, weeks or months) of specificity, intensity and volume of training to achieve peak levels of fitness for the most important competitions. So the answer to the question is "yes." Your clients need to do both. You should design your clients' programs so that sometimes they are working on endurance, and sometimes they are working on strength. The best way to do that is an organized system of periodization.

As you probably know, periodization organizes a training program into different phases, each one devoted to different goals. The theory of periodization evolved from Hans Selye's basic theory of adaptation to stress, which he called general adaptation syndrome. Selye theorized that when subjected to the stress of training three things happen: (1) the shock or alarm phase, in which the athlete experiences soreness, stiffness and the usual work-out-related aches and pains (2) the resistance phase, also called supercompensation, in which the athlete gets stronger and (3) the third phase, maladaptation, what most of us would call overtraining. Obviously, that's the one we want to avoid. The idea of periodization is to do just that by taking the body right up to the precipice without sending it over the edge.

When you think about training, after all, it is sort of like walking near the edge of a cliff. You're always trying to get as close to the edge (pushing the body to adapt) as you can without going over (overtraining or injury).

The specifics of periodization are beyond the scope of this principle. The idea, however, is to vary your routines so that you not only avoid injuries and overtraining, but maximize the gains from your training efforts. As a general rule, you can divide the year into several cycles of 3-4 months and assign different goals to each one. Consult any of the fine strength training books available for more specifics. Not only will your clients make more progress physically, you will help them avoid the mental staleness that often afflicts and discourages even the initially-motivated people.

Principle #48: Periodize your clients' programs.

 You're no slouch.

I always joke, not only with clients, but on the air, that I'm going to start my own "posture posse," a group of us who go around and make sure everyone's got their shoulder blades pulled back and their pelvises level. If I see one more person at the mall walking like Quasimodo, someone's going to die! (Probably me from a stroke because I let things like this drive me nuts!) As I always say, many people who think they need to lose five pounds just need to stand up straight!

It should come as no surprise that most adults have some serious, shall we say, challenges when it comes to their posture. The one I notice most often is a severe anterior tilt to the shoulder. (Think about Quasimodo again.) That's no surprise, since most people spend so much time looking down at computers, clenching their teeth in traffic and otherwise cooperating with the forces of man and nature always conspiring to grind us into the ground.

People are always amazed at how much flatter their stomachs appear when they work on correcting their swaybacked posture. It's an automatic feel-good when you show them. Sometimes their hamstrings are so tight that it's hard for them to maintain without a lot of conscious effort, but that's a good opportunity for you to remind them how important hamstring flexibility is, right?

While you're at it, make sure that you teach them by example; that is, it's more than a good idea to make sure you're not slouching when you see clients. In Principle #12, we discussed being a carrier of enthusiasm, and one of the best ways to convey enthusiasm is through your body language. It's a challenge at times to stand up straight and walk with a spring in your step when you feel like the dog's dinner, say after a long day of training clients. But if your mouth says "high energy," but your posture says "I'm beat," I don't have to tell you which one has the louder voice.

Just by way of review, you should adhere to the following checklist of posture points:

- Head floating on your spinal column, not hanging forward
- Ribcage lifted, with four-finger space between bottom of your ribcage and the top of your pelvis
- "Bones together"—my shorthand for tightening the transverse abdominis by trying to squeeze the iliac crests together so they meet under the umbilicus
- Pelvis level—imagine the top of your pelvis is a bucket and make sure nothing can spill out over the top
- Knees pointing forward, like headlights
- Ankles straight, not collapsing
- Feet pointing straight ahead, not turning out

It's not just "posturing." It really makes a difference, not only in terms of functionality, but also confident attitude. Pass it on!

Principle #49: Make your posture an example for your clients.

#50   *Excuse me, but do you mind if I make a suggestion?*

Sometimes knowledge can be a curse. In fact, one version of hell is knowing more than almost everyone else in the room, and not being able to say anything. If it's obvious that the other people in the room not only don't know what they should know because they are actively, even enthusiastically, demonstrating their ignorance, then silence can be torture!

I should know: I'm in this situation every single time I work out in any gym or health club. The things I see would scare a battalion of Navy Seals. I know those guys aren't afraid of anything, but trust me, when it comes to exercise, there are some very frightening things going on every day.

You see older women with such bad posture their heads appear to be growing out of the center of their chests trying to do lat pulldowns behind the head. You see young guys, egged on by their training buddies, attempting one-rep max bench presses and arching their backs so much that the areas of their bodies contacting the bench could be measured in microns. You see people using machines in ways their designers couldn't have imagined after a 3-day LSD binge. I could go on. I do, in my head, and sometimes on the radio, but NEVER to any of the afore-mentioned offenders. I don't say a word, even if it appears that the person is about to kill himself.

I saw a commercial recently for a product designed for people who wear glasses and don't want to buy prescription sunglasses. It is a little set of magnifying lens that fit on the inside of regular sunglasses, thereby transforming them into, I guess for a lack of a better phrase, reading sunglasses. In the ad, a rather annoying woman with a chirpy voice approaches people trying to read on chaise lounges by the pool and gives them a little spiel on how stupid they look trying to read with both regular glasses and sunglasses. And the first time I saw it, I thought "Thanks for sharing, but who asked you?"

The same thing applies to you in the gym. No one, I mean NO ONE, is interested in your suggestions, no matter how smart you are, no matter how knowledgeable you are, and no matter how right you are in this particular case. You will just be resented as an annoying busybody, which is I'm sure not what you are looking for.

Principle #50: Never be the officious intermeddler.

#51   *Because I said so!*

In my experience, there are some exercises that almost everyone hates, at least at first. (Leg curls come to mind.) Eventually, most clients get over their distaste for exercises they originally despise. That's because in the beginning some exercises are more awkward than others, and remember, that most of our clients are high-achievers who want to excel at everything.

There are some exercises, though, that they will always just hate. When you say it's time to do that exercise, you can see the enthusiasm evaporate like perspiration on a hot, desert day. They do the horrid thing, but grudgingly, and sometimes even moving on to another exercise they like, won't bring back the alacrity with which you started the workout.

Sometimes clients can be like picky-eating toddlers: they will go for months liking, or at least appearing to like, an exercise, then suddenly you hear "I hate dumbbell row." Huh? Where did that come from? More important, what should you do about it?

Let's say a client tells you, "I hate that stupid dumbbell pullover thingie that you've been having me do, and I don't want to do it anymore." I suggest that before addressing the issue with your client, you take a step back and ask several key questions:

Why does your client hate the exercise?

If it's that issue of awkwardness while mastering a new movement, see if you can coax him into hanging on a little longer. Explain that motor skills are a complex choreography, involving the firing of specific motor units in a specific order, and that it takes about 20,000 repetitions to get any level of competence. If the issue isn't initial awkwardness, perhaps it's your client's particular biomechanics. Are you doing the exercise on a bench that doesn't fit his body? Once I had a client who hated dumbbell rows. I found that when I moved to a bench that was lower to the ground, the discomfort that precipitated the dread of dumbbell row disappeared (try saying that fast three times).

Why did you include the exercise in your client's routine?

If you put the dumbbell pullover in your client's routine to work the lower part of his trapezius and pull down on his neck, I salute you. Most adults need that desperately. If you don't know why you put the exercise in the routine, now's the time to figure that out. Once you know that, you'll know whether you can simply eliminate it or whether you need to find a substitute exercise.

Are there other exercises that would accomplish the same objective?

In the case of the pullover, you can substitute a straight-armed lat pushdown. The dumb-bell row can work the same muscle groups as the lat pulldown, at least at a gross anatomy level, and vice versa. Be creative, and remember that one reason you get the big bucks is that you can figure out things like this.

Principle #51: If a client really hates an exercise, find an alternative.

 Wow! Cool stereo! Let me just turn it on and play... mmm... which CD do I want to hear?

The fact that our clients trust us enough to invite us into their lives is gratifying. The fact that they invite us into their homes is downright amazing. I have a famous client who I first met on-line. After a couple of e-mails had passed between us, he suggested we talk on the phone. After that, he suggested I come to his house. When we knew each other better, after six months or so of one-on-one workouts, I asked him whether he thought it was a good idea to invite someone you met on-line to your house. "Didn't you worry that I might be nuts?" He said that he trusted his instincts after talking to me on the phone. Actually, what he said was "I can always tell whether someone's nuts after I talk to him on the phone." And even knowing that, he invited me over anyway. Go figure.

I guess I wondered about that, not only because of the personal safety issues in-volved with inviting a stranger into the home, but simply because a person's home is his castle. When you're in a person's castle, you should act like it. Don't go around touching everything and picking it up, unless you are auditioning for the part of cleaning lady. Don't turn on the TV or the stereo without asking. In short, pretend you're five years old and visiting your fussy grandmother's house and don't touch anything.

Another suggestion: if your client gives you something to drink, ask if you need to use a coaster before just putting the glass on the table. Chances are the answer will be no, but the question will be appreciated.

I include pets in the category of client's property, so make sure you watch out for them if need be. Most of the clients I see just leave the door open for me to let myself in while they are warming up. One house features three frisky dogs who are constantly trying to escape. I've got to make sure they don't sneak by me when I'm coming in.

One more word to the wise: you never know when the client might have a twisted sense of humor like me and fill the medicine cabinet with marbles just to catch nosy visitors who might be snooping around in there. Avoid being a victim of similar mischief by not sticking your nose where it doesn't belong.

Principle #52: Respect your client's property.

 C'mon, any fool can plainly see. . .

When I was in college, with lots of time for navel-gazing and other exercises involving "pure" thinking, I took a lot of philosophy courses. I loved philosophy, but I concede that sometimes it's not the most practical subject. In one class, epistemology, we spent hours debating whether all the material objects that we perceived in the room might flash out of existence if and when we closed our eyes. (No wonder all the engineering and business majors dropped the course the first week.) Another similarly abstract topic involving perception was the meaning of color. For example, as you read the word 'purple,' you get a picture in your mind's eye of what that means, but is that necessarily the same picture I have in my mind? Of course not. But, wait a second, isn't it obvious what the word 'purple' means? No. It's not. That's what we're saying in this principle. It's not obvious, and the thing is the very word 'obvious' itself is just like the word 'purple': it means different things to different people.

I think that many of us in the fitness profession forget how oblivious most of the members of the public are to the information that we live and breathe all day long. It's not because, in my opinion, as some like to say, that most people are stupid. Most people are not stupid. They are distracted. They have way too much on their plates, both literally and figuratively, the former often due to the latter. In other words, they are trying to do too many things, and are constantly playing catch-up, which keeps them from knowing what they need to know about exercise and nutrition. Don't assume that "everybody knows" how often they need to exercise, at what intensity and for how long, or that they need to eat five servings a day of fruits and vegetables. Yes, I know that you can't swing a dead cat without seeing an article or a news report about exercise and nutrition, but I also know that people hear selectively. They miss a lot of this information because they think it doesn't effect them, or the consciously avoid it because it reminds them of something else they need to do, when they barely have time to scratch their heads every day.

The tricky thing is to make sure you tell clients and potential clients what they need to know without appearing to talk down to them. The way to navigate these waters is with the most effective oars of all: communication and empathy. Practice effective listening, and you'll learn shortly what your clients know and what information they need from you.

Principle #53: Don't assume that "it's obvious."

 Look at me! Look at me!

We used to think chin-ups were a great test of strength and fitness, but now we realize that heavier people, even those who might be strong, lean and healthy, are distinctly disadvantaged in this test. Still, many people think that the number of chin-ups or pull-ups you can do, is a measure of your fitness. I have a client who works out in her basement, where there are some steel beams. When I first started going there, I used to always do a couple of chin-ups on the beams, just for fun. (I would have done more, but the sharp edges of that beam kind of dug into my hands.) After a while I realized that maybe this sort of thing looked like showboating to her. After all, most women, even those who have worked out for a while can't even do one chin-up. She couldn't. It turns out she was amused by this habit, but not everyone would take it that way, I'm quite sure.

I know I sound like a broken record (for those of you born before 1980 who don't know what I mean, ask your parents or grandparents), but I don't think I can remind you of what I'm about to say enough. The people who hire trainers, especially professional, well-educated, well-qualified trainers, tend to be high-achieving and at times perfectionistic. The last thing they want from the person they are paying to help them get in shape and feel good about themselves is to hear how someone else is doing better than they are, even if it's true.

Forgive this rather unsavory analogy, but I think it applies: when a call girl shows up at a ritzy hotel for a "date" with a "client," she is careful to pretend that he is the only man in the world, and certainly the only man she's ever been with. That's what I read anyway, and I think it's a good model for us. When we're with a client, we need to pretend that he or she is our only client. He or she is—at least for the time that you're there. Keeping this in mind will convey the impression that you are as focused as you need to be to provide the level of service that you are determined to deliver.

Principle #54: Don't compare your clients to each other (or to yourself).

#55   ***Of course, sugar and fat have never passed these lips.***

Isn't it funny the way that so many clients think that we fitness professionals never eat "bad" foods? Once I was at a client's birthday party enjoying a huge hunk of gooey cake—MMMM—when suddenly I was nearly blinded by a barrage of flashes going off right in my face. Was I finally being struck by lightening after all these years of predicting it? (As in "if I blow off my cardio again, will God strike me dead.") Obviously, it was nothing that dramatic. It was simply several dozen people who wanted to preserve the event, Teri eating cake, on film. They squealed with glee, "Oh, I can't believe I got a picture of you eating that!" You'd think they were photographing Haley's Comet or something! The assumption among most people who call my radio show is that my eating cake happens about as rarely, but they are wrong. Granted, I don't eat sugary, fatty treats often, but I do on occasion. I also like to drink wine with dinner and eat candy at the movies. People are thunderstruck to hear these facts about me. I shudder to imagine what they would have thought if they had been with me at the National Sporting Goods Show one year. I had just witnessed a group of lean, sculpted exercisers perform an energetic step routine at the Reebok booth, only to see them outside moments later smoking like stoves. It turns out they were dancers. They were probably smoking to control their weight, but regardless, it even surprised me a little and I'm hard to shock.

We all fall short from time to time of the ideal, be it the fitness ideal, the parent ideal, or the worker ideal. You need to make sure your clients understand that you know this fact. It's a barrier to effective coaching to have them view you as sitting up on a lofty perch, Dr. Laura-like, lecturing them from above.

> **Principle #55: Demystify yourself and the whole process of being fit, and health will seem more attainable to your clients.**

 #56   ***I could try using the two-pounders, I guess.***

We want all of our clients to be superstars, people that we can not only point out as paragons of fitness virtue, but who also are delighted with themselves. Sometimes in our zeal to help them get there as soon as possible, we may overestimate their ability just a tad. It reminds of the time my husband facetiously suggested that someday he could set the world record in the marathon by decreasing his time 30 minutes per year until he got just under two hours; you know, the first year, he runs it in 4:30, then 4:00, then 3:30, then 3:00, then 2:30. . . you get the idea. Let me answer your unspoken question, Dear

Reader: Of course it's impossible! He knows it and he's joking. It's no joke, though, when we decide that a client should be able to progress up some arbitrarily derived linear master plan that we've got in our heads. "MMM. . .let's see now. . . he's using 15s for his flat dumbbell press now, and it's not *that* hard, so next week he can go up to the 20s, and the following week the 25s. Cool!" Perhaps this is an exaggeration, and perhaps some of our clients are capable of such prodigious progress, but most are not. The fact is that progress is rarely linear, and you have to be flexible enough to recognize that every single one of us gets stronger and leaner at his own pace. Not only are genetics a factor, but so are factors that change day to day, such as fatigue, emotional stress, hormone levels, dehydration, and sleep patterns.

You're always better off underestimating your client's ability rather than overestimating it. Recall that training is a process of breaking down tissue so that it can rebuild in a stronger version of its former self. Consequently, you are always walking along that perilous line between progress and injury, whether it's your own training or the training program you've designed for your clients. We want our clients to view exercise and good nutrition as lifelong activities, things they are committed to and that come as naturally as brushing their teeth, not things they do until they "get in shape," only to revert to their old couch-potato ways. Given that fact, err on the side of conservatism. Baby steps are good. You won't get there as fast, but you'll probably get there without having to take any prolonged layoffs due to injuries.

One thing you'll learn quickly: clients will surprise you. The ones that you think will make progress very fast may take forever to recover from a difficult workout. Some that appear frail and feeble are like one of those cartoon chickens who swallow a couple of cartoon megavitamins and burst out ready to open a can of whup-ass on everybody. Enjoy the surprises as they unfold. Sometimes it's a wild ride.

Principle #56: Be realistic about your client's ability.

 ### Let me get this straight. You WANTED to do the workout, but the mean aliens abducted you anyway?

Lots of excuses for not doing workouts are lame. Mine, yours, everyone's are. Some people hire personal trainers because they realize that they make too many excuses and they need someone to impose a little discipline on their lives.

Since we know that, I guess there is a strong temptation to look askance at clients when they explain why they didn't do the workouts we've assigned them as homework. It's good to keep them honest by hanging that continual threat over their heads, and more importantly, in the backs of their minds. Not wanting to get "the look" will keep them accountable and may give them the added push they need to stay motivated on those days when they're starting to wonder "what's the point?".

Sometimes a client will commence with the excuses the minute we make contact, either in person or by phone. It's sort of a pre-emptive strike kind of thing. "Before you ask me about it, I didn't ride my stationary bike last night. When I got home, my basement was flooded and I spent all night bailing it out! By the time I got done, I had to take a shower and go to work!" Some of the excuses are very creative, I must say. No, I'm joking: the fact is, my clients never lie to me, and I never lie to them. I think that if your relationship with your clients isn't based on mutual trust then you are never going to ascend to the level of excellence that you should demand of yourself.

If you discover that a client is giving a line of BS about things he committed to do, it's time to have a serious talk about commitment and trust. The coach-client relationship is in this way like a marriage: If he can't trust you enough to tell you the truth, you should probably move on. In the meantime, assume he's being honest and try to encourage him to do better next time.

Principle #57: Give your client the benefit of the doubt.

 Of course, he's a political weasel and a slimeball! Wake up and smell the coffee!

People who listen to my radio program know that I have strong opinions about almost everything, especially politics. Some clients find that discussing politics or other potentially inflammatory matters is enjoyable. If so, I'm more than willing to oblige, but while I don't hesitate to talk about these things on the air with perfect strangers, I do hesitate to do so with clients, at least until I know them extremely well and know for sure that these conversations won't damage our relationship or in any way interfere with what we're trying to accomplish.

As I said, some clients enjoy talking about politics. I have one client who likes to have CNN on during her workouts, and she'll draw energy from watching those reports. The more infuriated she gets, the stronger she gets! In her case, these conversations aren't a distraction, and since we tend to agree on most things, there's no chance of getting into a shouting match. That would definitely put a crimp in our workout!

It's not only issues of serious import that can be distracting. Once when I was practicing law, I was involved in a real estate deal that involved my traveling to meet with my company's new partners. They picked me up at the airport and took me to breakfast. That was my first, and I hope my last, exposure to grits. As I stirred the horrid-looking things, imagining alternative uses other than eating (wallpaper paste springs to mind), one of my charming hosts piped up, "Did you see 'Real People' last night? That show is so funny!" For those of you who don't remember 'Real People,' or who are lucky enough to have blocked it out, it was the great-grandfather of all those "World's Funniest" shows that have afflicted television in recent years. I disliked it (just as much as I dislike its successors), but I had to smile politely and say "I missed that." The truth was I never missed it: I never saw it, and I never missed it!

A good way to avoid running into trouble is to let your client take the lead in the conversation. That way you won't say something offensive, or if you do, at least it will be on purpose!

> **Principle #58: Steer clear of issues that might be a distraction to your client's goals.**

 #59   *I'm afraid there is the matter of my fee. . .*

I, like you, can probably think of at least one type of professional that shows up at somebody's house and then leaves with a wad of cash, but I don't think that those folks would be characterized as health professionals. (I know, I know, I made the analogy earlier in Principle #54, but I intended it to be limited to that one specific point.) So why do so many personal trainers seem to think it's a great way to do business? Of course, I am being a bit facetious, but seriously, not only do I find this billing system, if you can call it that, unprofessional, I think it potentially could cause a tremendous loss of income for a lot of trainers, and even increase the chances of their being sued.

Like all professionals, personal trainers need to have a professional billing system. Otherwise, I see four potential problems:

Unprofessional Impression

Accepting money at the beginning of a session is very distracting to what you are there to do and diminishes the impression your client has of you as a health professional. Your doctor doesn't ask you for money when you're sitting there in the examining room, does he? No, someone else handles that, so that your relationship remains, for lack of a better word, pure. Collecting money during your sessions reinforces the belief that he or she should treat you like a manicurist, a massage therapist or a hairdresser. What happens if you drive 20 miles to a client's house for your session and are told that he doesn't have any checks in his checkbook, and asks to "pay you next time?" What impact will that have on your focus during the session?

Lost Income

Second, there's the issue of lost income. How are you going to be compensated for your time if somebody cancels at the last minute if you're not going to be paid until you go there? Some of you may think you'll be able to collect for canceled sessions from clients who cancel at the last minute, but you've got a better chance sprouting wings and flying than you do of getting clients to pay you under those circumstances. On the other hand, if you've billed a client at the beginning of the month for all the sessions that month and you have a firm written twenty-four hour cancellation policy, then it will be easy—or if not easy, easier—for you to be compensated for this lost time. And remember, a personal trainer's time and knowledge are his stock in trade. That's why it's very important that you be compensated for late cancellations. When you block out time for clients, you can't commit that time to someone else. It's gone forever. So if you don't get paid, your income will suffer dramatically. Monthly billings in advance eliminate this problem automatically.

Gives Clients a Hammer to Use on You

Before I address this problem, I want to preface it with something very important: sometimes, as much as I try to keep her locked up, my inner lawyer gets out, so bear with me. The overwhelming majority of your clients are going to be wonderful, honest people who would not dream of taking advantage of you. Your relationships with all your clients should be based on Commitment, Integrity and Trust, and I'm sure that they will be. Once in a while though, you might run into a bad apple, so it's important that I tell you this because it may not be immediately obvious: clients who owe you money have a built-in incentive to find reasons to sue you. Here's how it could happen: A client owes you several hundred dollars for previous training sessions. When you press him for it, he suddenly discovers this horrible pain in his back that he NEVER had until he started working out with you. He doesn't want to talk to his lawyer, he explains, but money being as tight as it is, he might have to—medical bills are so expensive, and he also owes you that several hundred dollars. Of course, if you're willing to forget what he owes you, he's willing to forget the whole thing. He just doesn't see that he has any choice, he explains pitifully. Of course, you lose this deadbeat as a client—maybe you could refer him to your "favorite" competitor—but in the meantime you're out that income. If you bill clients monthly, and not allow them to get behind, you eliminate the temptation for someone to stiff you, using the threat of a lawsuit as a hammer.

Cancellations

I alluded earlier to a late cancellation policy, and I urge you to have one. What do I mean by that? I mean if clients do not notify you of a cancellation within twenty-four hours, they will be billed for the session. Some trainers have a specific cancellation fee; that is, they don't bill clients for the entire missed session if cancellation is given within a certain time frame. You could consider something along those lines if you think it is fair. But, whatever you do, have a firm written policy on cancellation and make sure every client understands it from the beginning. There's nothing more detrimental and souring to a relationship between you and a client than arguing about cancellations and whether they're going to pay you for them.

Principle #59: Have clear, written billing policies.

 #60   *Maybe I need to be hypnotized.*

Once your client hires you, if you work it right, he will start to view you as an authority on all matters relating to his health and fitness. That's great! As their resource person on these matters, they will seek your advice when they need help with something. They will ask you for referrals for other professionals who can help them make more progress. When they do, you need to be able to oblige.

Not only do you want to make yourself a one-stop shop for fitness, you want to get your name out there. You see, it's not only for the benefit of your clients that you want to develop a network. It's a great way to stir up a little buzz for you and your business. People who go to dietitians and massage therapists will probably be the same sort of people that you'd like to have as clients. Think about it: they are striving to be their best and they are willing to make some effort to get there. You need to get your name to these people and let them know what you can do!

Here's a short, and by no means comprehensive, list of the professionals who should be in your Rolodex:

- Massage therapist
- Chiropractor
- Registered dietician
- Orthopedic physician

If you don't currently know any skilled people in these categories, start looking for them today. Ask your clients, friends, relatives, and anyone else who might be able to put you on to someone special. Then contact this person and tell them that you are interested in reciprocal referrals. You might even want to consider offering a discount to new clients who call and use the referring party's name. That's a great way to build goodwill, both with the new client and the person who referred him.

Between the benefit of knowing that your clients are being well-served by someone who considers you a friend and a source of referrals and the benefit of having your name mentioned by more and more of the best professionals in town, this is a win-win!

> ### Principle #60: Develop a network of allied professionals.

 ### MMM. . .Let me just check that time and temperature.

You should want to talk to your clients as often as possible, although I understand that sometimes at the end of a long training day, the last thing you want to do is talk on the phone. I don't deny that. All I'm saying is this: If you are going to call anyone, call your clients first.

It's a no-brainer, or should be if you have the right attitude. Your clients should come first. Call them before you call your long-lost college roommate, your friends, or even your mother. (She'll understand when you call her later.) It's simply a matter of priorities.

You are probably assuming that I say this because it goes along with my whole clients-first philosophy, and you are partially right. I want you to be in the frame of mind that causes you to think of returning your clients' calls first without my suggesting it. That's the right thing to do.

If that's not enough reason for you, consider this: if you call your clients back ASAP, you might save yourself a lot of time. What if you don't call a client back until several hours after you have already prepared a series of high-intensity workouts for him? Feeling tremendously satisfied after typing them up, you call and your client tells you he was in the emergency room earlier that day getting his broken leg set in a cast. "I guess I won't be working out, at least no legs, for a few weeks," he sighs. Don't you wish you had known that before you spent several hours preparing that high-intensity leg workout for the next day?

> ### Principle #61: Return client calls first.

#62   *Emergency 911.*

Do you know whether your house is in an area served by 911? "Duh, Ter," you may be thinking, "EVERY place is served by 911!" If you think that, you probably think every health club provides free towels to members. Of course, the consequences of one erroneous assumption might leave you dripping wet and embarrassed. If you're wrong about 911, wet (as in your pants) and embarrassed might be the best thing we can say about you if things break bad.

Not every place in the country is served by 911. I hope you never have to find out, but the time to do so, is not when your client is writhing on the floor, gasping for breath.

The first time you go to a new workout location, ask your client two questions: "Where is the phone?" and "Is this area served by 911?" He may look askance and say something like "Are you going to push me until I have a stroke or something?" That's your opportunity to display your high degree of professionalism by explaining that while you've never had to call 911 yet (assuming that's true), if you do, you want to be ready.

Thinking about emergency situations is a good opportunity to evaluate the workout area for potential dangers, and then modify it to eliminate them. Remove slippery area rugs and other trip-and-fall causers.

Principle #62: Have an emergency plan for every location.

 #63   ***Well, that was after my ex-husband came back to the trailer with the ax.***

Do you think of yourself as an authority figure? Well, you are, at least to your clients. I've found that one of the biggest challenges of being an authority figure is that you have to be "on" all the time; that is, even if you don't feel terrific, you have to radiate enthusiasm and energy. A related point is that even if you have a lot on your mind, you have to put it aside and concentrate on your clients.

Your clients think of you as the person leading them up the path to optimum performance. You are the one who is going to help them identify, and then overcome, the barriers and obstacles that are keeping them from being their best. They trust that you know the way. If you come off like an emotional basket case, that's going to be a tough sell.

I was slogging away on the elliptical trainer once when I struck up a conversation with the woman next to me on another elliptical trainer. As we chatted, I noticed that she had very beautiful fingernails. Eventually, she told me what she did for a living: she is a manicurist. Of course. I commented on her nails, and she said "Yes, I have to keep them looking good. No one is going to want to go to a manicurist who has crummy looking nails." Exactly.

Perhaps you're familiar with the minor controversy in our own profession about whether clubs should hire plus-size (I think that's the PC term) instructors. Regardless of your position on this issue, the salient point is that some people believe there is an inherent inconsistency between someone overweight, or who is perceived to be overweight, assisting others in reaching their ideal weight.

"But, Ter," I can hear you protesting, "I'm not overweight. I've got a six-pack to die for, and you could break a 2 x 4 on my firm, tight rear end." Fine. My congratulations to you, but I don't care how great your body looks if your life is a shambles, and your clients KNOW your life is a shambles, they won't view you as the person to help them become their best. Now, if your goal is just to be a glorified spotter and rep-counter, maybe you can skip this principle, but I don't think you want to settle for that.

Principle #63: Keep your personal problems to yourself.

 Excuse me, Officer, could you please take me home? I'll try not to drip too much on the seat.

I grew up in Phoenix, Arizona, a place that is sunny about 340 days a year. On most days, if the TV weather guy wanted to take the day off, he could just re-run the previous day's forecast and no one would have known the difference. I guess that's why it wasn't until I moved to the Midwest that I understood that weather prediction actually involved some skill. In fact, these forecasts are frequently wrong! Imagine that.

Of course, it wasn't just watching the weather reports that taught me about the unpredictability of Midwestern weather. I got a very personal and very embarrassing lesson in this subject one morning during a pre-breakfast run. It was summer, so I set out especially early to avoid the heat. The sky was clear, but the air felt a little heavy. Unaware of what this heaviness might mean, off I went. I was about 2 miles from my apartment when suddenly I looked up and saw what could have been a black curtain appear to draw across the sky. The blackness engulfed the blue sky, spreading like black ink spilled on a pale carpet. Then came the thunder and lightening. I was in the middle of horrific thunderstorm. Fortunately, I was near a mall. I hid soaked and shivering under the overhanging roof of a nearby restaurant until a police car happened by. Humiliated, but desperate and without any better idea, I ran out from under the roof, waving my arms to attract attention. The police officer, obviously amused, instructed me to get into the car and he took me home. I'm sure that I provided some entertainment around the doughnut shop for the next week or so. For my part, I learned an important lesson about the unpredictability of weather.

Take-home message here: Allow extra time to get where you need to go when the weather is iffy. Since weather can be so unpredictable, carry a portable phone to let clients know when you might be late.

Principle #64: Prepare for weather emergencies.

 Baseball pitching? It's my specialty.

You should be proud of yourself for spending the requisite time and effort to become a genuine health professional by getting an education. After all, in our unregulated industry, some boneheads just get a few business cards printed up, strap on the thong and they're ready to go. Since you are a professional, you should be the first one to know that no one person has the right combination of personality, education and practical experience to help everyone reach their goals.

I have a colleague who used to be a major league baseball pitcher. When an acquaintance called and asked if I could help her college-age son, a high school superstar on scholarship, prepare for baseball season, I thought of him immediately. I know something about the rotator cuff, and I love baseball. Of course, I could help him. I realized, though, that I couldn't help him as much as my colleague. He not only knows about anatomy, physiology and biomechanics, he's actually been a baseball player. My friend appreciated my honesty, which enhanced my reputation as a professional who seeks to do what is in the interest of clients.

Keep in mind that it isn't just sport-specific things that might make one trainer a better fit with a client than another. It's also personality and person style. For some clients, it might be gender. I have a client, a male, who once told me that there was no way for all the tea in China that he could be trained by another guy. It would feel more like competition to him. You might encounter people with the same preferences. Don't take it personally. Rather, consider it an opportunity to work with the clients you can help the most.

Principle #65: Don't assume that you are the right trainer for everyone.

 That's enough of that for one day.

In the beginning of your career, you will probably be tempted to try to do many things in every session. Eventually, you'll learn that you can effectively do about seven exercises max and do them well. And that's the point: you can't do everything and do everything well.

You are much better off planning to do fewer exercises well rather than trying to do everything and end up blowing off half the exercises that you planned, or even worse rushing trying to fit everything in.

If you do this right, remember, you will be working with this client for a while, so there will be plenty of time to teach them lots of different exercises. You don't need to rush through anything.

It takes time to instruct a novice in the proper way to do a squat, a lat pulldown or a bench press. I think sometimes because we work out so often, we forget how difficult it is for a beginner to master movements that are second nature to us. While it will be tempting to think "Oh, she's got it. Let's move on," resist that voice. It's tempting you down the wrong path, the path of rationalization and sloppiness. You're not after "good enough." You're looking for mastery.

Principle #66: Halfway is no way.

 Because I said so.

Good personal trainers are teachers (refer to Principle #2). You want to leave your clients more knowledgeable about fitness and nutrition than they were when you found them. At a higher level of abstraction, you want them to know more about anatomy and physiology, too.

I'm not saying that you need to get into the MEGO level of detail (Makes Eyes Glaze Over). Trainers who want to prove that they've studied their anatomy books and are the smartest people in the room are not trying to explain anything. They are trying to show-off and making horses' asses of themselves in the process. As I always say, you don't have to understand internal combustion to be able to drive a car. Still, you want to give them a general idea of why you have included certain exercises in their programs. Not only because you're trying to teach them, but also because you will get a better result if you do.

Think about your own workouts. When do you get a better workout: when you make a mental connection between the exercises your doing and why you're doing them or when you just go through the motions? A no-brainer.

Clients will be more focused, more committed and more compliant in every aspect of their programs if you tell them not only how to do an exercise, but why they are doing it.

Principle #67: Explain the why as well as the how.

 Tragedy in the forest preserve. Film at 11.

Earlier I mentioned my embarrassing story of getting caught in the thunderstorm (refer to Principle #64). Now, imagine the same story, only this time, it's me *with* a client. That would have been a thousand times worse. Not only would it have been really embarrassing, perhaps my client would have gotten hurt. Suppose he slipped on the wet pavement, or stepped in a hole scrambling for shelter from the thunder and lightening. I can think of dozens of bad things that could have happened because we were in an outdoor location away from any forms of communication.

You know that sometimes apparently healthy people drop dead during exercise for no obvious or apparent reason. Earlier I told you about my friend and training partner running with her husband at a high school track. This apparently healthy, lean, non-smoking 35 year-old went down completely unexpectedly as a result of an undiagnosed enlarged heart. Fortunately for my friend and her husband, the location was not that remote, although she should have had her cordless phone along. There were people around and one of them did have a phone, averting what might have been a tragedy.

I don't want to sound like some sort of finger wagging nervous Nellie, but it's just not a good idea to take clients into locations where you have no control over what happens. Often that's a perfect definition of the great outdoors. Weather, animals, miscreants of every description may await you. Even though it might be fun to go walking out in nature, I'm not sure that the risk outweighs the benefits.

Principle #68: Use extreme caution about taking your client into remote locations.

 To leave a message, stand on top of a high mountain and yell really loud.

I suspect that it has always been extremely frustrating when you want to talk to someone and you can't. I'll bet Abigail Adams was frustrated a lot when she and her husband John were separated while he was working on establishing our cool country. There were lots of things that she needed to tell him, as we can see in her letters.

I think you can make an argument, though, that it's much more frustrating today because in the olden days people didn't expect to reach anyone that they had something to tell within a few minutes or even seconds. People DO expect that today, thanks to that the double-edged sword that is technology.

Even if people can't talk to you, they expect to be able to leave you a message. Many people, I happen to be one of them, have terminated their business relationships with professionals because of an inability to at least leave a message. I used to have a dentist, note "used to" as in ex-dentist, whose phone was not answered from 12 noon-1 PM because "it's lunch time." When I pointed out the availability of inexpensive voice mail systems, the dentist responded that he didn't see the need for that. Patients like me could just call back. But, as I explained to him when I asked him to transfer my records to another, more technologically-hip, dentist, patients shouldn't have to call back. When we take the time during our busy days to call to make an appointment, we want to check that item off our "To do" list. Under his system, it remains undone until they decide to re-open. I don't think so! I am quite sure that most of your clients and the people who eventually become clients will feel the same way.

Principle #69: Be reachable.

It took forever to boot up, 20 seconds—NO LIE!

The meaning of that word "TIMELY" has changed in the last ten years or so. Recently I was in a retail store and I noticed that every time someone bought something with a credit card, the woman behind the cash register said "That will be right up." When I got up to the register to pay for my purchases, also with a credit card, she said the same thing. "Don't you get sick of saying that?" I asked, and she replied, "Yes, but people are so impatient these days." And of course, we are. Technology has completely changed everyone's expectations about how long things should take. If you're thinking "This effects me how" here's how: you need to be responsive to your clients, and these days "responsive" means being reachable (refer to Principle #69) and being reachable virtually 24 hours a day, 7 days a week.

Today there's no excuse not to have your phone answered in a professional way, given the affordability and availability of voice mail. Pagers are also cheap and available. These days people expect to be able to reach everyone at any time, or to at least be able to leave a message for that person. We're all too busy to get into a run-around. We want to call and check that off our list.

Do you ever get sick of having your pager on and getting client calls at any time of day? Maybe, but remember your goal is to run a profitable personal training business, and that means being responsive to clients. That's all that matters to them.

> **Principle #70: Understand the new meaning of "timely."**

Do you eat with that mouth?

Recently a man in Michigan was ticketed and tried for swearing in public. I'm sure you heard about this case because, even if you tried, you couldn't escape it. I think a nuclear warhead could have been dropped on New York City, and this still would have been the lead story for some reason.

The case seems ridiculous to me because it doesn't seem like a police matter. I understand, though, the feelings of those who say that something should be done about the coarseness of our general discourse these days. Words that used to be heard only on the deck of a tramp steamer are now used on network television. While I have an extremely high offensive threshold, I also recognize that some people find swearing extremely offensive, and they will assume that the person speaking in such a low manner is some sort of guttersnipe. Definitely not the image you're working hard to create.

It may not seem fair, but it's true: people judge us by superficial things, including the way we speak. One reason I find appealing about the play "My Fair Lady" is its underlying premise that a person's station in life can be determined by his speech patterns and the words he uses.

I'm sure that you will have your party manners with you every time you're with a client, but just in case you have any doubts, here's my suggestion: don't say anything in front of your clients that you wouldn't say in front of your mother, at least in the beginning. After you've known them 5 or 10 years, I'll leave it up to you whether to let your guard down from time to time.

> **Principle #71: Watch your language.**

 #72   *I'm the one giving the standing O.*

When I first began my personal training business, I worked with some clients in a gym and some in their homes. The gym was the one where I worked out, and was a fine place with a few notable exceptions. One such exception was a well-known member who made no secret of the fact that she was a devotee of steroids and cosmetic surgery. Not that she needed to say anything: she could have fit in just fine in a circus side-show, not only due to her freakish appearance, but also her boisterous, rude behavior. She especially resented anyone who knew more about physiology than her, which was just about everyone, but especially me. Once when I was working with a client, and applauding a particularly great set of squats, she loudly bellowed that I looked "like an idiot standing there clapping."

She was half right: I was standing there clapping. I still do sometimes. It's usually not something contrived. I just get so excited at seeing someone reach back and get that extra rep, that it's the natural thing to do.

There are many ways to praise your clients. Of course, just telling them "good job" after a workout is something you should do on a regular basis. Sending cards, e-mail or snail mail variety, when they've had a particularly good exercise week is always appreciated. When a client tells you how proud he is that he did the treadmill five days this week, just as you discussed, that client is due for a little gift, in my book. Your clients will cherish these little momentos, no matter how inexpensive. They will be badges of honor representing their pride in achievement and your recognition of how hard they are trying to be their best.

Principle #72: Praise their successes.

 ### Is it ok if I go to the bathroom?

I know I said that we should consider one of our responsibilities teaching our clients, but I don't think we should be like kindergarten teachers, giving our clients permission to go to the bathroom and letting them know when it's ok to get a drink of water. Clients don't necessarily see it that way. Many, even most, will assume that they need your permission for these things, and just about everything else that happens during your sessions.

While it is desirable for clients to take direction from you during your sessions and to view you as an authority figure as a general matter, you don't want them thinking they have to be trying to do sets of heavy squats with their bladders nearly bursting because they are afraid of disrupting the rhythm of the workout.

In your first session, which should be an orientation of sorts, you should explain that the client doesn't need your permission to get a drink of water, to go to the bathroom or to do anything else. If frequent interruptions become a problem—say, if a client insists on taking every phone call that might come in during your session, even calls from telephone magazine salespeople—then it's time to have a talk about how these unscheduled breaks are major barriers to the progress he hired you to help him achieve. During this talk, your objective should not be to tell your client how you would not tolerate any more interruptions. Rather, it should be to explain that if the interruptions continue, he won't get as much from his sessions. If he's ok with that, you should be, too.

Most clients don't want any interruptions during their supervised workouts. The point is that some can't be avoided, either for physical reasons or for reasons involving issues in the client's life. It's up to the client to decide when to take a break.

Principle #73: Explain who is really in charge.

#74 ***Today I want you to work on doing every repetition slowly and under control.***

You and your client have worked together to formulate short-term, intermediate and long-term goals for him. I'm suggesting that you micro-focus and set goals for every workout. Starting each session with specific goals for that day creates a natural partition between the mental chatter that afflicts your client and diminishes his concentration during the rest of the day.

The goals you set don't have to be complicated. In fact, simple goals are the best. Here are some examples of goals that I have set for specific workouts:

- Concentrate on contracting the opposing muscle group from the one you're working

- Make sure you do the negative part of each repetition slowly. Aim for a count of 6-8.

- Let's work on being completely present with every thing we do today. Stay completely in the present moment and don't think of anything beyond the present moment.

- Perfect form for this exercise means keeping your elbows in contact with your rib cage, so focus on that on every rep.

You get the idea. Giving clients a focal point not only improves form and effectiveness, it makes the workout mentally refreshing, almost a form of meditation.

Principle #74: Have goals for every workout.

 #75 ***Just put your hand into this box and pull.***

Recently a listener to my radio program sent me an article from a local paper. It was about working out at home, and purported to demonstrate the fact that you don't have to spend a lot of money on equipment to do strength training effectively. One guy interviewed in the article had constructed a bench out of some milk cartons and other junk he found in the garage. He made some bizarre-sounding dumbbells out of old auto parts, and a barbell out of a used axle from a truck. Innovative, and as long as he's going to use that equipment only for his own workouts, fine by me. If he wants to use it with clients, we've got a serious problem.

Commercial equipment is designed to withstand the rigors of normal use. It is tested to make sure it can. Contrast some cobbled together thing that might fall apart right in the middle of a repetition and land indelicately right on your client's pretty face. Or some homemade bench that might collapse when your slightly-heavier than lithe client puts his ample keyster on it. Kaboom! Eight point five on the Richter scale! And, by the way, have you met my lawyer?

The same cautionary note applies to using unconventional household objects as makeshift "weights." I've seen lots of articles in those annoying "women's" magazines suggesting that women use soup cans as weights. (I wonder how many IQ points I lost by reading one of those publications.) I understand their desire to encourage women to work out at home with what they have at hand (no pun intended), I think they need to reconsider this suggestion. Unlike commercial dumbbells, which are designed to fit a hand, cans are not. They can very easily slip out of the hand and land right on the toe before you can say "mmm...mmm.. good."

Save your creativity for designing workouts, and use high-quality well-maintained commercial equipment when you work with clients.

Principle #75: Don't use homemade equipment.

 ### *Regis and Kathi Lee—Oh, yeah, I LOVE them!*

Not really, but I had a client who did, and so we used to watch them during workouts. Not really intently, of course, but they would be on the tube in the workout area. Sometimes people, hearing about this, would say "how can you allow that? Doesn't she get distracted?" No, not really, at least not during her sets, but only because I kept her focused when she needed to be focused. I didn't mind having the TV on because I could tell that it made her more comfortable. I never shared my opinion of the show or its hosts.

Some clients like to listen to music when they work out, be it big band, classical, or heavy metal. Whatever your client finds motivating, you should embrace with enthusiasm. Failing that, you should tolerate it, even if it makes you grind your teeth and feel like hurling. If your client likes it, he's really not interested in your commentary about how much it sucks. Dummy up about that, and be grateful for the extra motivation.

Another aspect of control will be the ambient temperature. Learn to layer so that you can anticipate and be comfortable in almost any temperature. Some clients will sweat like pigs when it's only 70 degrees, while others are cold when it's 78. Lots of workout areas are in basements, which can be damp and therefore feel cold, even on comfortable days. If you wear a sweatshirt over a T-shirt over a workout outfit, you can peel off what you don't need or leave on what you do. You'll get to know which homes are kept cold and which are as comfortable to you as your own, so dressing the part will get easier.

Principle #76: Let your client control the environment.

 Here's that stuff about turtles that you wanted for your grandson.

My clients are the greatest people on the planet, and there's almost nothing they'd ask me to do that I would not do, or at least try to, if it were in any way within my power. I've gotten information about turtles from my vet for a client's grandson, dropped off a cherished photo at a photo place for restoration, and helped carry a 150-pound dog up the stairs. Really. I didn't do any of these things because I could bill for them. I didn't and I wouldn't dream of taking money from a client for doing a favor, even one that took a long time. I'm not, as you may be thinking, talking only about favors unrelated to working out. I don't charge them extra for preparing summaries of their workouts or other workout-related work I might do on my own time on their behalves.

Does this conflict with Principle #14, in which I suggested that you make sure you don't undervalue your service? This Principle is not only not in conflict with the suggestion in Principle #14, it's an integral part of it. Here's how: one of the reasons that your clients will be willing to pay you the big bucks is that you provide unsurpassed customer service. Most people would rather pay a little more and get excellent service, than pay an ostensibly low price and then be nickel and dimed to death for every little extra.

I was talking to my friend the massage therapist who told me that she knew other therapists who charged significantly less than she, but who charged her clients extra for every single little thing. "You want some Tiger Balm on that sore muscle? That's an extra $3." I think in this context you can see how disruptive this is to the client-practitioner relationship.

Principle #77: Don't bill your clients for everything you do for them.

#78 *Touch my firm derriere. I dare you.*

As you know, the trainer-client relationship is a personal one. In many cases, your clients will view you as the only person to whom they can reveal their real, vulnerable selves. During workouts, they can let their guards down and be themselves. They don't have to pretend to be the strong, I-have-everything-under-control professionals, Supermoms, or Masters of the Universe that they must be nearly every other waking hour.

When someone opens himself completely to you, that puts you in a unique position of trust and responsibility. That's Level 3 (refer to Principle # 9). Remember, though, you must keep a professional distance between you and your clients. Ethical professionals understand that it is inappropriate to become romantically involved with clients. I assume when I say this that I'm talking about a trainer and client who are both single and unencumbered. Any other sort of romantic involvement is so far out in left field that I don't even want to imagine the moral minefield that presents. Even if there are no moral issues, though, there is the issue of effectiveness.

Your effectiveness depends on your ability to be an objective, albeit compassionate, authority figure. You must be governed by thinking and logic, not emotion. If you become too emotionally involved with your clients, you won't be capable of providing them with the type of coaching they deserve.

You should limit touching to the clinical sort of touching that a doctor or a professional massage therapist would find appropriate, such as using a finger to cue the muscle or muscle group that you want them to mentally envision. Only in rare occasions should you have them touch you. I can think of only one that is definitely appropriate: having them touch your body so they can feel a muscular contraction on a particular exercise. The most notable example of this type of client-touches-Teri is demonstrating how to depress the scapula during a lat pulldown. Otherwise, maintain a professional distance, literally and figuratively.

Principle #78: Keep your relationships with clients friendly, but professional.

Anything he can do, I can do better.

Recently my stockbroker of nearly twenty years, Jim, changed firms. I expected, and shortly thereafter, did receive a phone call from the guy—let's call him "Mr. X"— at his old firm who had been assigned the task of keeping clients from switching firms. Given our long association, one might conclude that I am pretty happy with Jim and his performance. (I am.) You'd think this salient fact might have entered the mind of Mr. X, but apparently it didn't. He decided that the best strategy for retaining my account would be to engage in a little trash talk about Jim. Bad move. This is what you call a lose-lose situation: his chances of getting my account did not improve one bit (they were always zero), but he made himself look bad in the process.

As we all know, personal training is an unregulated industry. Those of us devoted to elevating the professionalism of the field have our work cut out for us, there's no doubt. Everywhere you look you see imbeciles masquerading as professionals and making all of us look bad in the process. It's perfectly fine for me to say this in general terms, here in this book, or on television or radio. It would be a completely different story, though, if I were talking about a specific trainer. No matter how stupid or incompetent another trainer is, if you point it out, it makes you look bad, envious, petty, and negative. I strongly recommend you avoid doing it at all costs, especially if you're trying to take away his clients.

In fact, you should take a cue from the legal profession on this one. If you know a person already has a trainer, you should refrain from any discussions with him about his trainer, his program or any related matter. If the client becomes unhappy with his trainer, maybe he'll call you. Maybe he won't. Regardless, if you run around trying to steal other trainers' clients you do several things, all of which are bad for you: first, you make enemies, and in this cold, cruel world, none of us needs more enemies; and you make yourself look bad in the eyes of the client, even is he agrees to come over to your side. I've always wondered how these ditzy homewrecker bimbos delude themselves into believing that even though their "great guys" cheated on their former wives, they won't cheat on them. Yeah, right. The client you steal today could be stolen right back tomorrow, and you'd have nothing to say about it.

A word to those of you who work for personal training businesses, and decide to go out on your own and take "your" clients with you. These clients signed on, not because of you, but because of the reputation of the personal training business. Ethics and standards dictate the you negotiate a buy-out with your former employer, which all reasonable employers would be happy to do. This obligation exists even if clients you worked with while employed by another firm call you after you leave. If ethics and standards aren't sufficient motivation for you, consider the fact that in most communities, the fitness community is a small one. What goes around, comes around.

Principle #79: Don't steal other trainers' clients.

 Gluttony, lust, and not carrying business cards.

In my opinion, there should be a special place in hell for those who don't carry business cards. Don't you find it annoying to have some bonehead give you a big piece of notebook paper, or even worse an old gum wrapper or a grody receipt, with his phone number written on it?

You should view every social occasion as an opportunity to spread the word about what you can do to improve the health and fitness of every human being on earth. These gatherings are your chance to make a positive and professional first impression. The ripped piece of notebook paper is not the way to do that.

You just never know when you are going to run into someone who can help you. Sitting on an airplane, on line at the movies, standing in the produce section. I personally have done some serious networking in the most unlikely places. You just never know when someone you've given your card to might call you. Months, even years later, you'll hear from someone, all because your card fit into a Rolodex. Try doing that with a giant piece of paper.

Your business card is the only essential marketing piece that you need. If you work it right, it can function as a mini-brochure. Don't take that as a suggestion that you make it real busy and hard to read. Include essential information, plus a catchy tagline if you have one.

Cautionary note: Recently a friend showed me a business card that a personal trainer had given him. It featured a deeply-tanned, greased up torso with an awesome set of six-pack-dominant abs, and thick, well-defined pecs and arms. He said "Have you ever considered having a card like this?" I explained that I hadn't, and then suggested that he note one thing: the fact that there were no initials after the guy's name. I congratulate him for not appending any phony initials to try to pretend he had credentials, but I also fault him for circulating a card that suggests a million dollar body is all you need, even if you have a two-cent brain. Would a doctor or physical therapist have a card like this? I don't think so. Please don't make the same mistake.

Principle #80: Always carry business cards.

 I'm glad that you asked me that question.

Have you ever noticed how when certain politicians, the skillful ones in my opinion, will always greet a loaded question with a response like that. "Matt, I'm so glad you asked me about those illegal campaign contributions." Right. Those political weasels want questions about their sordid little schemes like we all want a railroad spike through the head and everybody knows it. Isn't that one reason for the corrosive cynicism that afflicts our society?

Earlier I mentioned that you need to de-mystify the whole process of getting fit (refer to Principle #55). I've also suggested that you avoid the cardinal sin of taking yourself too seriously (refer to Principle # 10). This Principle is about both of those things.

Some people have such a huge investment in being "experts" that they are afraid to admit that they don't know, or remember, everything. Stop and think, though: don't you think people see through this act? Smart ones do anyway. They know in their own lives that there are many questions that they can't answer, and most of them will be "experts," or at least professionals in their own fields.

The best thing to do when you are asked a question that you can't answer is to admit that you don't know. As Mark Twain said of doing the right thing, you will gratify some people and astonish the rest. That's not the end of the story, though (refer to Principle #82).

Principle #81: If you don't know, say so.

#82   *I'll get back to you on that.*

The corollary to Principle #81 is that if you don't know something you know where to find out. While no reasonable person can expect a professional to know, or even to remember, everything, no reasonable professional can expect to be respected if he doesn't know where to find out.

I can remember screaming at one of my professors in graduate school after an exam. (Imagine what fun it was to have me in class. Now that I'm a college teacher myself, I'm sure I'll get some of that back.) I was furious because he expected us to regurgitate the list of enzymes in the Kreb's cycle. As I said, "why clutter up our brains with things we can always look up? That's not thinking!!"

Most of the questions clients ask will involve a little of both, looking up information and thinking, as in figuring out how it specifically applies to them. As for the first one, make sure that you look for information from credible sources. Supermarket tabloid stories about the dramatic effects of the latest fat-burning supplement are amusing, but they usually aren't based on good science. In fact, you must be extremely skeptical of any story in the press about exercise and nutrition. Unfortunately, most members of the media couldn't pass statistics at gunpoint, and they tend to be very lazy. So, someone, usually someone with a hidden agenda, sends out a press release and they print it almost verbatim, treating a valid, replicable study in the same way that they'd treat the results of 3 guys in a bar comparing their training diaries. Don't rely on the popular press, print or broadcast, for your fitness information. Instead, get your information from current textbooks or peer-reviewed journals, such as *Medicine and Science in Sports and Exercise* or the *ACSM Health and Fitness Journal*, both published by ACSM, *The Physician and Sports Medicine*, and *IDEA Personal Trainer*. There are many other good publications out there, but there are, sadly, many more bad ones. The Internet is a very rich source of information, but you must be skeptical of what you find there. Healthy skepticism in these matters won't ever let you down.

Principle #82: Know where to look it up.

#83   *I'm on a break.*

Recently I was talking to a client about time. She is typical of my clients, extremely successful and high-achieving, a partner in a major accounting firm. She was relating her most recent week, which featured her being in 6 cities in 6 days. Exhausted? You think? Definitely. I commiserated with her, and let her unload a little. After a sufficient venting period had expired, I broached the topic of over-scheduling. "Maybe you're a bit overbooked. I know that sometimes you can't help it, but maybe once things settle down a bit, you could devote some time to thinking about how you might avoid being in this situation in the future." She thought about it for a minute, and then said "You know, it never seems like you're overbooking yourself when you make all these plans. The reality of it doesn't hit you until you're in the middle of it, and by then, it's too late to change anything!"

So true, and worth noting for all of us who are tempted to work 24/7. In case you hadn't noticed, personal training is a challenging job, both physically and mentally. If I asked you at the end of a long training day whether you had more time in your schedule to take on some new clients, you'd probably say "Are you nuts? I'm half-dead here!" You need to stay in touch with that feeling of completely wrung-out exhaustion when you're tempted to add more responsibilities to your day. It's like running a marathon (or I'm told, childbirth): immediately after the event, you say to yourself "This was the most damn painful thing I've ever been stupid enough to do, and I've learned my lesson." Weeks or months later, after the stress fractures have healed and you can barely see the place where they put the IV, you think "MMM. . .maybe I could have a personal record in the marathon this time," and the pain and misery is a faint memory, overshadowed by your enthusiasm for a victory you can almost taste. It's the same thing with taking on too many clients and too many projects. You can easily become blinded by thoughts of being able to reach so many more people, and then there's the extra revenue coming in. This blindness makes you oblivious to the fact that you are heading for a crash, a real burn-out disasterfest.

The other problem with overbooking yourself is that you will have very little flexibility to accommodate client requests for schedule changes, and that will inhibit your ability to provide excellent customer service. Make it a point to schedule at least a couple of hours every day for yourself, not including the time you spend on your own workout. You'll be glad you did.

Principle #83: Take time for yourself.

#84   *You're in good hands.*

Liability insurance is like your spare tire: you hope you never have to use it, but you certainly are glad it's there when you need it. I don't have a lot to say about liability insurance, except this: get it, and don't talk to a single client or potential client until you have it. Not that liability insurance will protect you from getting sued. It will protect you if you ARE sued, though, and that's the important thing. In addition, most potential clients are going to ask you if you have liability insurance. The reason they will is not because they don't have confidence in you, but because everyone realizes that no matter how smart or how careful people are, accidents happen. That's what insurance is for. If and when an accident happens, your insurance is there to protect you and to compensate anyone who may have been injured as a result of the accident. Let's face it: exercise can be dangerous and with all those heavy objects swinging through free space and things on the floor gyms are minefields. So given that fact, only a real beanbag would avoid having liability insurance. Think about it: you're a safe driver, but you still have auto insurance, right? Of course you do.

There are other people who might be interested in whether you have liability insurance or not. If you are lucky enough to be a personal trainer who is allowed to come into a gym or a health club as an outside trainer, the owners will at a minimum insist that you provide them with evidence of liability insurance.

Principle #84: Maintain your liability insurance.

 #85   *Gotta go.*

Sometimes when you and your client finish a session, he'll look pretty fried, especially if it was an especially intense workout. You congratulate him on a job well done, and you're on your way. That's no problem, unless what the client is exhibiting is something a little more than just normal post-workout fatigue. For example, if you are working with someone particularly obese and de-conditioned, and you push him a little too hard, he might become light-headed. Sometimes even those who aren't obese or particularly de-conditioned get light-headed. There are lots of reasons that this could happen. Low blood sugar, dehydration, recent illness, lack of sleep and stress are just a few that spring to mind. Obviously, we as personal trainers cannot diagnose the cause of light-headedness or any similar malady, but the main thing I want you to know is that if this happens, stay with your client until he feels better. Offer to get him some water, or call someone for him if he lives alone. In short, do whatever you would want someone to do for you or a loved one in a similar situation.

There are other situations when you'll want to stay with your client until he's back on an even keel. I told you that clients will often share very personal, and sometimes painful, feelings with you. You might be the only person with whom they can release this pain. It's not unusual in these situations for clients to cry. I don't want you to be frightened or intimidated by this sort of thing. It's a normal reaction, and is usually quite cathartic, and therefore, good for your client. Your job is to be empathetic, ask if there is anything you can do to help, and most of all, stay with him until he's gotten it back together. I can usually bring a client back to normal with one of my especially lame and stupid jokes. Some who have heard my jokes might suggest that no one who has one inflicted on him is better off, but at least they aren't still crying!

Principle #85: Never leave a client worse off than when you found him.

 Yes, no, maybe.

We've been over the fact that you shouldn't pretend to know the answers to questions when you don't (refer to Principle #81). The way to handle these inquiries is to know where to find the answer (refer to Principle #82). The important thing is to be responsive, and to be responsive and truthful.

Responding doesn't always mean agreeing to do what you're asked. Sometimes it will mean referring your client to a competent, knowledgeable professional like yourself (refer to Principle #60). Sometimes it will mean telling your client that despite your best efforts you couldn't find an answer. Let's hope you don't get many questions like that, but you may, and the important thing is to be authentic. The personal trainer-client relationship is one of integrity and trust, like all important relationships, so whatever you do, tell the truth.

A brief word about this honesty thing: I don't know if you have been as distressed as I have by stories in the popular press about how "everyone lies," suggesting that lying is nothing more than a strategy for getting through the many dicey situations in which we all find ourselves periodically. I find these stories more appalling evidence of the decline in standards that is sending our society into a slough of social pathology. People who run around ringing their hands wondering how we ended up with all of these social problems should remember that it's better to light one candle than to sit and curse the darkness.

What does this have to do with your relationship with your client? I want you to understand that it's NOT "normal" or appropriate to be dishonest, even to protect yourself from embarrassment or to attempt to gain some advantage over someone or for any of the other gazillion reasons (actually rationalizations) that dissemblers use to justify their mendacity. If you don't want to be honest because it's the right thing to do, do it for the cynical reason: if you always tell the truth, you don't have to have such a good memory.

If your client asks you for information or help, take care of him as soon as you can, as well as you can, and always as authentically as you can.

> **Principle #86: Always respond to client requests promptly and truthfully.**

 #87 *A mind is a terrible thing to waste.*

No one knows how much it sucks to go back to school as an adult as one who has done it. That would be me. When I decided to change careers, I needed to go back to school for my master's in Exercise Science. School wasn't the walk in the park that I remembered from my undergrad days. Actually, I think even law school was easier because it was the only thing I was doing at the time. When you go back to school after several year's absence, often you're dragging the baggage of a job, a family and lots of other things that weigh a lot more than a backpack full of textbooks.

I guess it's this time-challenged-adult thing that makes people distinctly unenthusiastic about going back to school, or even taking continuing education classes. While I understand those feelings, I know that you will be making a big mistake if you don't take advantage of all the terrific continuing education opportunities available today.

It's a funny thing about knowledge. It doesn't change, and as long as you use the stuff you know every day in your work, you don't forget it. I see three major problems with just letting things stay where they are as far as your knowledge base is concerned. First, what you know you know, but that's all. Exercise physiology is relatively a young discipline. It didn't begin until the late 1960's, and so research is continuing to advance the frontiers of knowledge. You've got to keep up. Second, attending workshops and classes revives your enthusiasm and freshens your perspective. If you just keep getting by on the same old information presented in the same old way your presentation to clients will become like one of those stagnant ponds on those nature TV shows, just sitting there fermenting and getting even more stagnant with every passing day. You want to be more like a free-flowing stream, teaming with new ideas and new ways of sharing them. Third, if you don't attend any workshops, conferences and classes, you won't do as much effective networking. You need to interact with other fitness professionals, to find out what they have to offer and to share your programs with them. It is from a healthy, dynamic Rolodex that many a fine career has been built.

If you're still not convinced, remember that your continuing certification probably requires you to do it anyway.

Principle #87: Take advantage of continuing education opportunities.

 Only the best is good enough.

A friend told me a story about two boys who decided to dig a hole all the way to the center of the earth. As they were digging, two older boys came along and asked what they were doing. When the first two boys told them, the older boys burst out laughing. "You'll never be able to do that!!" And the older boys went on their way. The youngsters dug all day and got exhausted in the process. At the end of the day, resigned to the fact that the older boys were right, they abandoned the project. As they sat in silence, feeling a bit discouraged, one boy held up a jar full of spiders, worms, and assorted insects, and said to the other, "well, we didn't make it, but look at all the cool things we found along the way!"

This Principle refers to one focal point: being your best. That should be your goal every day, and that's what goals are for, to make sure you start digging. View every day as an opportunity to be better than the day before. Even if you don't make it, the effort itself will make it possible for you to do things you didn't think you could do. Your clients will be the lucky beneficiaries of your pursuit of excellence, and so will you.

Living a life of contribution is a journey, one that you should strive to enjoy every single day. Of course it won't be easy. If it were, every bonehead would be doing it. By definition, the pursuit of excellence means doing more than is expected and doing so with alacrity and empathy for your clients.

Strive for excellence, not perfection, and enjoy the journey!

Principle #88: Be determined to exceed expectations every day.

CONCLUDING THOUGHTS

I hope that the principles presented in this book help you in your daily quest to be the very best personal trainer you can be. I also hope that reading them will inspire you to think of more. If it does, I look forward to hearing from you. Until then, be your best!

Teri is available for workshops, keynote addresses and lifestyle coaching. To contact her, write:

Teri O'Brien
Teri O'Brien Fitness Systems, Inc.
106 W. Calendar Court, #81
La Grange, IL 60525

Phone: 888-523-5326

E-mail: teri@teriobrien.com

Internet: www.teriobrien.com